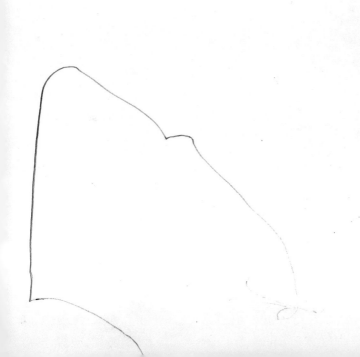

Choices in Childbirth

Choices in Childbirth

Dr. Silvia Feldman

Publishers · GROSSET & DUNLAP · New York
A FILMWAYS COMPANY

The publishers gratefully acknowledge permission to reprint material on the following pages:

p. 36 *The Supermarket Handbook* by Nikki and David Goldbeck. Copyright © 1973, 1976 by Nikki and David Goldbeck. Used by permission of New American Library.

p. 72 *New Miracles of Childbirth* by Elliott H. McCleary. Copyright © 1974 by Elliot H. McCleary. Used by permission of David McKay Company.

p. 75 *The Feeling Child* by Arthur Janov. Copyright © 1973 by Arthur Janov. Used by permission of Simon & Schuster.

Copyright©1978 by Dr. Silvia Feldman
All rights reserved
Published simultaneously in Canada
Library of Congress catalog card number: 77-95181
ISBN: 0-448-14524-3 (hardcover edition)
ISBN: 0-448-14525-1 (paperback edition)
1979 PRINTING
Printed in the United States of America

For my mother Ethel, who helped so many women.
And my dear husband Eli, who helped me.

Acknowledgments

Researching *Choices in Childbirth* was an exciting adventure in post-graduate education. Warm thanks to the many people who took so much time and trouble to help me find my way.

I am particularly indebted to Dr. Mieczyslaw Finster, professor of Anesthesiology at Columbia University's College of Physicians and Surgeons in New York, and to Doris Haire, president of the Foundation for Maternal and Child Health in New York. Dr. Finster and Ms. Haire spent many hours with me, painstakingly reviewing the material about drugs, anesthesias and medical practices to make sure the presentation was accurate and fairly balanced. For any errors which remain, the responsibility is mine.

Thanks to Dr. Stanley James, professor of Pediatrics, Obstetrics and Gynecology at the College of Physicians and Surgeons; Dr. Frederic Ettner of the American College of Home Obstetrics in Chicago; Dr. Yvonne Brackbill, graduate research professor, Department of Psychology and Department of Obstetrics and Gynecology at the University of Florida; Dr. Lewis Mehl, director of Research for the National Association of Parents and Professionals for Safe Alternatives in Childbirth; Dr. David and Mrs. Lee Stewart, co-directors of NAPSAC; Dr. Catherine De Angelis, director of Ambulatory Pediatric Service of the University of Wisconsin at Madison; Dr. Tom and Mrs. Gail Brewer. Each played an important role in helping me assess childbirth practices in the United States, while Marilyn Freedman, president of the Long Island, New York, chapter of ASPO, contributed her excellent program for physical fitness.

Many more doctors, midwives, nurses, childbirth educators and other health specialists also helped: Drs. Michael Bergman, Victor Berman, Eli Feldman, Robert Fitzgerald, Daniel Friedman, Lawrence Gartner, Joseph Hindman, Jacqueline Rose Hott, Ilan Israeli, Judith Kestenberg, David Kliot, and Jerry Maisel. Also Barb Barosa, Elisabeth Bing, Mary Cossman, Gay Courter, Sue and John Crockett, Peggy Drake, Andrea Eagan, Janet Epstein, Teddi Grauer, Janice Greene, Jay Hathaway, Lester Hazell, Betty Hosford, Sat Jwan Kaur Khalsa, Gladys Lipkin, Ruth Lubic,

Jeanine Parvati Medvin, Helen Miles, Doris Olson, Gail Peterson, Jane and Jim Pittenger, Janet Reinbrecht, Judith Roehner, Barbara Seaman, Jeanne Sommers, Anne Tebbit, Patsy Turrini, Fran Ventre, and Jayne Wiggins.

I am also thankful for the perceptive guidance of my editor, Sylvie Reice, and for the invaluable help of her assistant, Judith Brown.

I am grateful for the splendid cooperation of hospitals, nursing and midwifery organizations, alternative centers and childbirth organizations throughout the country. And to the many mothers who shared their childbirth experiences and their creative ideas and plans for improving American childbirth—a special thank you!

CONTENTS

Preface

Choices in Childbirth has turned out to be quite different from the book I initially planned. My original aim was simply to present birth today so the reader could make her own choice according to her own emotional and psychological needs. In the process of research, however, I learned that many complicated problems are involved both in making this choice and in carrying it through. As a result, I found myself stressing the pitfalls —the pain, problems, and risks—as well as emphasizing the clear possibilities for pleasure and fulfillment in the various choices.

If you want to avoid unpleasant facts, this book is not for you. If it disturbs you to learn that things can and do go wrong in childbirth, that there is considerable controversy among experts about how to prevent these problems and handle them when they do arise, you will be upset by what you read. However, this knowledge can be of invaluable assistance if you want to plan your childbirth rather than passively deal with it and "trust in fate and the doctor," as one woman I interviewed expressed it.

As a psychotherapist and marriage counselor, and mother of three girls, I have known for a long time how important a good childbirth is for happy family life. The childbirth experience affects not only mother and baby but the whole family as well. There have been such dramatic changes in the childbirth scene in the twelve years since I had my last child that I found myself exploring it with as much wonder, excitement, and surprise as any new mother. The new technology—electronic fetal monitors, stress tests, amniocentesis—and the newer methods of natural childbirth—Lamaze, Leboyer, Bradley—have revolutionized childbirth in America today.

The last decade has been characterized by two sharply opposed trends. The first is toward more aggressive medical intervention during pregnancy, labor, and delivery. The second is a countermovement to more family-centered hospital births and, most recently, to out-of-hospital settings such as childbearing centers and the mother's own home.

The experts are polarized into two camps. The new technologists are certain that extremists in the natural camp seek to return childbirth to the Dark Ages, and their opponents feel just as strongly that too much medical management is dehumanizing and violates what should be a joyful and fulfilling experience.

I believe it's important for every woman of childbearing age to be aware of this controversy, since it affects her life and future. While I lean in the direction of the "natural camp," I have made every effort to be thorough and fair in my presentation. I honestly believe that no one way is right for everyone! We are very different from one another in our psychological needs. Individual decisions must be made, every step of the way, that suit the person involved and achieve the goals she feels are most important.

Do you want to get through the birth experience with the least involvement and responsibility possible? Do you feel secure only when you're behaving in the traditional pattern? Do you want a doctor to lean on, a doctor who will tell you what to do and which way to go? Or do you want to participate in all decision making? What about your mate? How much—if at all—does he want to get involved? These are but a few of the many important personal factors that are essential to consider in making choices in childbirth.

An individual's personality is the result of all her previous life experiences. Genetic predisposition, her own birth and babyhood, her family's values and child-rearing practices, her social and neighborhood environment, her school experiences, her feelings about sex and her body, her work, her friends, and her marriage—all play a role in determining what she needs, wants, and is ready for when she becomes pregnant.

Experts of every persuasion agree, in theory, that a woman's personality must be considered in her childbirth choice. But paradoxically, they are convinced that their particular method is best for almost everyone! I have no one method to champion, and some experts are likely to be upset by my conclusions—especially when they don't agree with theirs.

Doctors who are convinced that the new advances in obstetric science are being misunderstood and unfairly criticized won't be happy with the section of this book that documents the risks that accompany the new technology. Obviously, many of these interventions are necessary and life-saving in special situations, but when they're abused, as too often they are, there are alarming disadvantages and side effects. Most traditional doctors feel it is up to the physician, not the patient, to decide when interventions are necessary. I believe that the woman must be fully informed and given the opportunity to decide for herself whether the benefits of a particular procedure outweigh the risks because she is the one who is stuck with the consequences!

Breast-feeding experts, too, may be disturbed that I pay so much attention to "combined feeding" (partial breast-feeding, supplemented by bottles and solids), since this practice frequently leads to termination of breast-feeding. However, I believe that partial breast-feeding is the solution many women want, and that it can work and provide the emotional satisfaction and closeness that breast-feeding bestows. But to make any decision about breast-feeding, a woman needs to know the disadvantages as well as the advantages of all feeding methods. Then she can select the one that suits her best, freely and with enthusiasm.

Home-birth advocates won't be too happy reading this book either. Some of them knowing how hard it is for young couples to find qualified assistance at home, are encouraging "do-it-yourself" childbirth in the belief that their specific education can prepare everyone for safe home birth. I don't share this optimism.

My research leads me to conclude that parents who plan a home birth need a properly prepared home environment and postpartum supports, as well as backup arrangements with doctors and hospitals should that infrequent emergency arise. Otherwise, I recommend spending the same energy to locate a childbearing center, a natural-childbirth enclave in a medical center, or a local doctor who is sympathetic enough to help you make exceptional hospital arrangements. If you have to go a distance to find such help, my research shows that it's worthwhile; the first few days are very important in establishing the mother-child relationship.

While writing this book, I have met so many friendly, helpful, open-hearted, and dedicated people of both points of view that I feel unhappy in advance knowing that some of them will be hurt, even outraged, by some of my conclusions. But I owe allegiance only to the people who are having babies. I believe that a full, straightforward presentation of all the facts will strengthen them. Shielding adults from unpleasant realities is no way to help them. With full confidence that the people who read this book are grown up, or fully prepared to be, I respectfully offer my work.

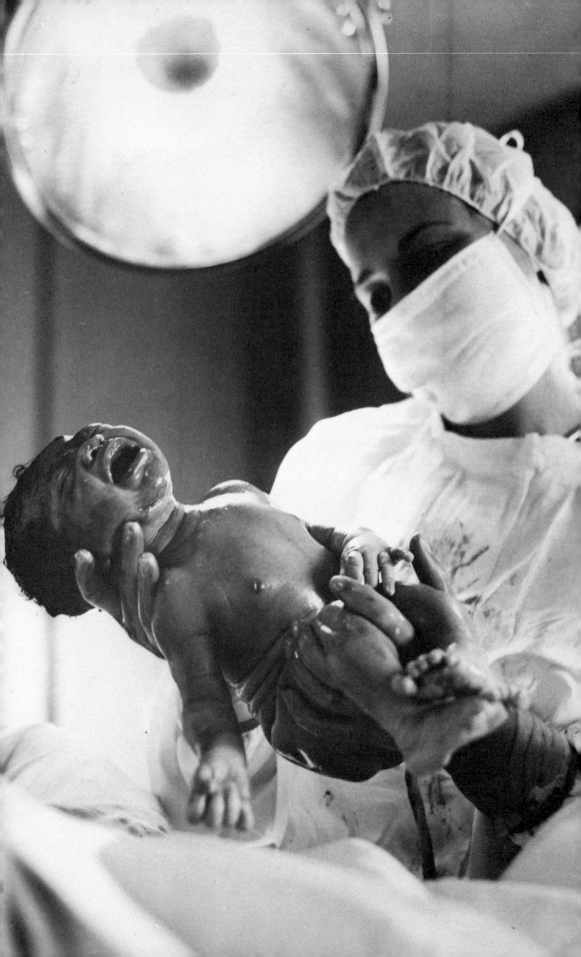

Introduction

More than three million babies were born in the United States last year. Each one had an experience many psychologists believe to be the most important in life.

While there is still controversy among experts about how much we human beings are affected by the birth experience, an increasing number are saying that it sets the pattern for later development that continues throughout our lives. Our attitudes toward ourselves and the world around us are connected with the way we first experienced our world as we came into it. Psychologists and neurologists are discovering that every early experience—in the womb, during birth, and into childhood—is recorded in the body and brain of a child and replayed through his or her life.

People who have had more positive birth experiences are easier to satisfy in infancy, more secure in childhood, and seem to be more optimistic about life when they are grown. Those who have trouble getting born seem to find trouble for the rest of their lives.

There is even some evidence of an association between a very difficult birth experience and subsequent mental illness. Of course, the usual consequences of birth trauma are rarely so serious or dramatic, but one large study reports a significant relationship between birth trauma and psychosis in later life when other negative factors, such as a family history of mental illness and poor early life experiences, also exist. In some cases, a subsequent mental illness could have been predicted years before it occurred.

Other consequences of difficult childbirth occur more frequently. These have adverse effects on the quality of family life, with mother-child, father-child, and marital relations the losers.

Childbirth experts believe that the way a woman feels emotionally and physically during pregnancy and delivery and the amount of contact she

(American College of Nurse-Midwives/Maternity Center Association)

has with her baby directly afterward strongly color her "motherliness"—her feelings about being a mother. Unfortunately, the American way of childbirth is insensitive to these feelings. Most civilized countries wouldn't think of routinely separating mothers and babies directly after birth (as we do) and keeping them apart merely to suit hospital practice. The mother's early experiences with her baby are thus made uncomfortable, clumsy, and unreal at exactly the time when her feelings should be allowed to bubble forth in an atmosphere of privacy and intimacy.

Before the birth of her own baby, the average American woman has little, if any, opportunity to hold, fondle, and care for an infant. Also, rarely does anyone speak to her candidly about how isolating and boring full-time motherhood can be. If the actual childbirth has been a frightening experience, if the hospitalization afterward has been upsetting, the unprepared mother is a prime candidate for depression after she returns home with her baby.

Postpartum depression is a nightmarish feeling about the new role and its responsibilities that just won't go away. A substantial number of American women suffer some symptoms of depression after childbirth, particularly with the first baby. Some fail to function altogether and need medication, supportive psychotherapy, separation from the baby—even hospitalization and shock treatment—before they can shake off feelings of terror and inadequacy and begin to manage on their own. Even a mild postpartum depression, lasting a few weeks, can leave such deep scars that the foundation of the early mother-child relationship is weakened.

It is not uncommon for women, later in life, to have total recall of those early, miserable days. Many trace later feelings of bitterness and disappointment in their roles as wives and mothers back to the first days at home with the new baby, when they felt overwhelmed, isolated, and unsupported.

Fathers, too, can experience serious stress while their wives are pregnant, during the child's birth, and in the first months of adjustment to the baby. Often, the behavior of the absentee father can be traced back to this period. Men who are encouraged to participate fully from the start, who attend preparatory classes, who accompany their wives through labor and delivery, and learn baby care at their bedsides in the hospital are much less likely to suffer these bad effects than those who are left out or absent themselves out of squeamishness or fear. For any member of the family—baby, mother, father, other children—stress during the childbirth experience can cause problems. Marital rifts, sibling rivalries, abusive parental behavior toward the children, and joyless, unhappy homes are some of the possible results.

It is very possible to prevent these unhappy consequences by preparing realistically for the whole childbirth year. While you are pregnant, or even before, is the practical time to think ahead to labor and delivery, to postpartum recuperation, to feeding and caring for the new baby, to rearrangement of your home to accommodate the new family member. And I suggest three major guidelines for this preparation. They are: *know yourself, know your options,* and *learn to communicate.*

The *first* important step for a woman who is becoming a mother is to explore her feelings about motherhood and childbirth. People are entitled to have the kind of childbirth experience that will best support them, that will be most gratifying and least stressful according to their *own* personalities and needs.

Second, become fully informed about your options, so that you can assess how much of what *you* need is indeed possible to obtain. What is childbirth "within the system" in your community? And is anything available "outside the system"? Are there nurse-midwife units in any of the large hospitals in your area? What about finding a doctor for home birth? What experiences have friends and neighbors had with these offbeat arrangements? Look into the safety and practicality of every kind of option that interests you—from traditional hospital stays to home birth.

Third, explore your neighborhood, family, and your own marital relationship to set up the kinds of postpartum supports that will make new motherhood happy and successful. Every new mother needs all the help she can get from family, friends, and neighbors to function at her best while she learns her new role.

This book makes it possible to plan a good childbirth for yourself on the basis of a realistic assessment of *your* emotional needs and on *your* informed choice. It helps you to choose between monitored and natural childbirth, to select from the many kinds of natural childbirth preparations, and between breast and bottle, or combined feeding. It offers the latest facts about nutrition, exercises to prepare for a normal childbirth and postpartum recuperation as well as for cesarean section. It extensively reviews studies about mother-infant bonding, about the advantages and disadvantages of drugs and anesthesia from both a physical and a psychological point of view, and it assesses all the available childbirth settings.

This book offers many practical tools and guidance to increase self-knowledge, to improve marital communication, to find sympathetic doctors and hospitals that will meet your needs. There is a carefully selected bibliography to help you in every area discussed. There is information about how to reach all the natural-childbirth, midwifery, breast-feeding, home-birth, and other organizations. In turn, they will help you locate neighborhood resources to support your own plans.

In many ways, the most important part of this book deals with your day-to-day life (and your husband's) after the baby comes. It is designed to help you get back on your feet with the least pain and the greatest pleasure possible, by candidly discussing the problems of the first six weeks, how to avoid postpartum depression, and how to deal with it if it develops, as a couple and an individual. An important preventive, you will learn, is establishing your supports in the community *before* the baby comes. All the presently available resources are critically evaluated to help you find what is best for you.

Step by step, *you* consider the possibilities and ask the right questions. As *you* arrange your childbirth, you will find that it's important to have a great deal of correct information, to know what you want, and to know how to ask for it sensibly and convincingly. Learning how to be an exception—something most of us hate to be in everyday life—may turn out to be the most important tool you will get from this book. It will help you to join the army of individual women, local groups, and national organizations that have begun to make fundamental changes to improve the childbirth experience of all women.

What is best for you—that is the focus and the message of this book. You do not have to trust to fate. Neither you do have to struggle alone, isolated and depressed, after the baby is born. May your childbirth experience be a rewarding, happy journey of self-discovery!

Part One:

BECOMING AWARE

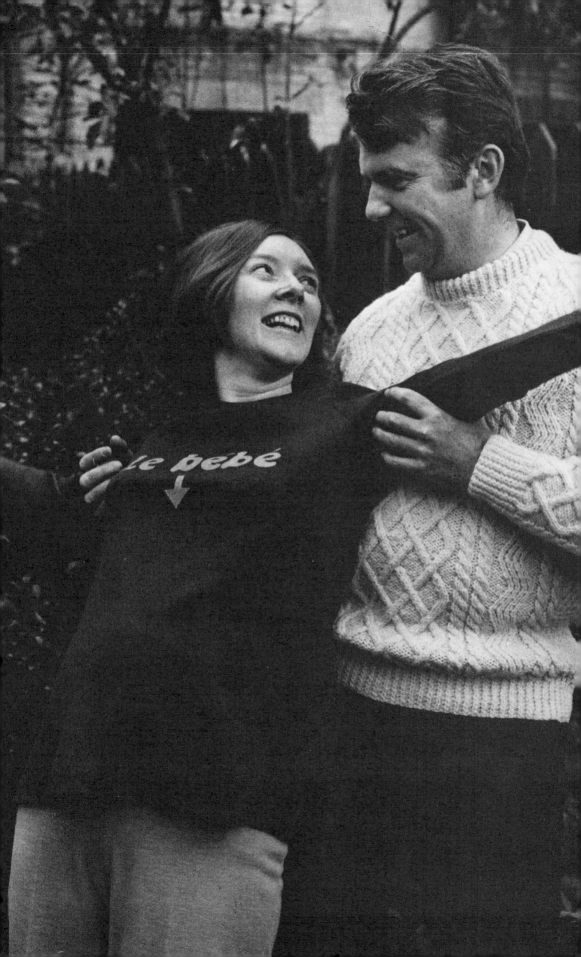

I

Widespread Ignorance about Childbirth

In some ways, having a first baby gets more complicated all the time. Once upon a time, generations of a family lived close together. Everyone knew the same doctor, the same local hospital. Sometimes babies were born at home, sometimes not, but always there was plenty of advice, emotional support, and practical help available. Young people became parents with strong familial support.

Then we all moved apart and away. Ignorance of baby care increased as family proximity and size decreased. "Ninety-nine percent of the mothers in my class have never seen a newborn baby before they take care of their own," says Helen Miles, director of Nursing and Health Programs of the Nassau County, New York, Red Cross.

Adding to the problem of inexperience is a conspiracy of silence among people who already are parents. Many had such a painful time in the early years that they loath to talk about it. That's really a shame; hearing about the bad as well as the good experiences would make young couples realize they should prepare for parenthood. Candid sharing of experiences has become as obsolescent as family and practical support.

These societal changes have led to unfortunate emotional consequences for new parents. Portpartum depression is frequent today, and disillusionment and resentment of parenthood are even more common. The seeds of future marital rifts and child abuse and neglect are planted in ignorance about what childbirth and child care are really like.

Young couples today rely too much for guidance on the first doctor they see. They tend not to seek additional sources of information about what to expect in the normal course of labor and delivery, what possible complications may arise, and how to secure the best possible hospital experience as well as the best home arrangements once they leave the

Most women feel at the peak of emotional and physical fitness during pregnancy. (Erika Stone)

hospital. Even in such important personal decisions as whether or not to breast-feed and whether or not to have natural childbirth, they are too influenced by their doctor's prejudices.

I think it is much wiser to get a broad spectrum of opinion first—to talk with other people who have had babies, to ask them questions about their hospital and postpartum experiences. You also can learn a lot about childbirth from documentary movies, television programs, and the many good books that are available. On page 251 you will find a wide range of resources as well as special books that will inform you in depth about each subject discussed in this book.

Many women refuse to ask questions or find answers on their own. Instead, they ask for—and get—glib assurances from their doctor that everything will come out all right. Unfortunately, they often find out that it doesn't.

RESISTANCE TO KNOWING

Why do so many young women resist getting information about child-birth? For most, it's because of a deep fear of giving birth. That fear can be conquered by facts that make childbirth a maturing rather than emo-tionally shattering experience. If childbirth education began in high school, women could take its normal stresses and strains in stride.

Dr. Daniel Friedman of Lawrence, New York, has done research on "parturiphobia," or fear of childbirth, among high-school girls. He has found that "the young girl absorbs from her elders and peers fearfully distorted accounts of labor and delivery." His study of fifteen-year-olds found that "58 percent already were afraid of childbirth, 72 percent pro-fessed no knowledge or had distorted concepts of childbirth." His con-clusion? "Fear is an all-pervasive factor of childbirth. Women are still concerned about suffering acute pain, undergoing serious body dam-age, or dying. Only a minority can accept the biological process for what it is. By the time they get to childbirth, they already have a phobia." Proper education and reconditioning are the methods he uses in his own practice to overcome this phobia. It's important to note that 250,000 babies were born to teenage mothers last year.

Fear is not the only reason women resist learning about childbirth. A typically American kind of carelessness can also be a cause. Adolescents blithely ignore the importance of caring for their bodies, which seem to thrive on a steady diet of soft drinks and junk foods. "The baby's going to grow no matter what you eat," one teenage mother-to-be recently told me. She is handling her anxiety by denying her pregnancy, including her responsibilities for proper diet and exercise. Fortunately, she is a minority, because she may learn the hard way that childbirth is just too important to blunder through.

Many older American women feel that they were inadequately prepared to take care of themselves or their new babies. "Why didn't anyone tell me how hard it is?" said one tearful mother, depressed when she thought she should be overjoyed. Another reported, "Giving birth itself was wonderful, but I feel very disappointed in my family and friends. They never told me what I was in for, and now none of them come around to help."

Yet childbirth experts who want to teach pregnant women the practicalities of child care find that many are hardly interested. They are so focused on themselves and "getting through" the birth that they don't want to hear about the problems that may come afterward. As Dr. Friedman observes, "If women were educated early enough not to be afraid of childbirth, they could better accept pre-, intra-, and postpartum education."

If you have postponed consideration of any aspect of the childbirth experience, now is the time to ask yourself *why.* The healthy, confident mother-to-be is full of curiosity, while the depressed and fearful one puts off learning, and get bored or agitated when the discussion turns to baby care. Facing the anxiety and overcoming it will free you to prepare properly for your new role. It is foolhardy to embark on such an important undertaking without thorough preparation.

HOW WOMEN REACT TO CHILDBIRTH

Social worker Patsy Turrini, of the Family Service Association of Nassau County, New York, recently studied the childbirth experiences of women in her community. Here is what she found:

Before the baby comes, women are afraid to ask questions of their doctors. None of the women interviewed doctors before selecting one. They had many unexplored feelings and fears, particularly about sex. (Some women felt guilty for having sex during pregnancy—others for refraining.) Most felt unprepared for what actually occurred at the hospital. They reported their doctor had told them "not to worry" and to "rely on him."

In labor and delivery, women were unsure when labor actually started and reported arguments with their doctors on the telephone about it. After a frantic trip to the hospital, the women were upset by admission procedures. They felt cut off from their husbands, dehumanized by "prepping" procedures (enemas, shaving). Unless Lamaze-trained (a course in prepared childbirth that entitles the husband to stay with his wife during labor and delivery), most women were left alone during most of labor, including "transition" (when the cervix fully dilates and the baby is descending), the hardest part of the labor. They reported vivid memories of isolation and terror, of being told they were "good" or "bad" by nurses. Those who were "knocked out" (by anesthesia) regretted the loss of memory afterward.

In the hospital, many women begged and cried to see their babies. (Many hospitals isolate babies in the nursery for up to twenty-four hours.) Frequently, there were fears that something was wrong with the baby. First experiences feeding the baby were frightening. Women were embarrassed to ask for help, and felt guilty for "peeking" (unwrapping their babies to look at them against nurses' orders). They worried about their other children at home, missed them and longed for them.

The return home was overjoying at first, but then there was a sudden onset of fear and feelings of helplessness. This was less acute if a grandmother was present to help. The most frightening experience was the inability to understand why the baby was crying. Nursing mothers felt most inadequate at these times. There were frequent feelings of rage at the baby. (Scars from these feelings lasted a long time.) Being restricted was very hard. The amount of fatigue was surprising. Visitors were perceived as a heavy burden. Physical pain and discomfort were common. The problem of isolation became worse as the baby grew and went on a regular schedule.

CHILDBIRTH THROUGHOUT THE WORLD

Today, more than 80 percent of the world's babies are born at home. Almost all births in the developing nations occur at home. In most industrialized nations the proportion of home births has steadily declined until their percentages of hospital births are almost as high as our own. The Netherlands remain the one industrialized country with a large proportion of home births. Even there home births are declining at the rate of about 3 percent a year, and they now constitute only 40 percent of total births. The Dutch government is presently concerned with the high expense of continuing a dual system of delivery.

Why have home births declined so rapidly? All over the world the tendency is to follow America's lead in hospital and technological childbirth. Social prestige in these countries is now associated with hospital birth, as it was in America in the early 1900s. Many European women today are asking for "modern" interventions, such as epidural anesthesia, where they have the choice and the money to pay for them.

There is one striking difference between American childbirth and childbirth in the rest of the world—midwives, not doctors, deliver most babies, except in the U.S. In developing countries these midwives are traditional village assistants, while in industrialized nations they are trained professionals, sometimes nurses. Where nurse-midwives practice there is a higher rate of technological intervention, while non-medical midwives tend to view childbirth as mostly a natural process, and turn over problem situations to the medical practitioner, usually a physician.

An American baby is more than twice as likely to die on the first day of birth as a Scandinavian or Japanese infant. And many people tend to believe it's because we interfere more with the natural process. The Netherlands, with a large home birth practice, has a lower infant mortality rate than we have. Has the movement to hospital birth and technological interventions been the reason for the low infant mortality In most industrialized countries?

Experts differ widely in their interpretation of the data. Advocates of the "American way of birth" believe these methods result in continual improvement. Partisans of home birth and natural childbirth maintain that improved infant survival is really the result of better hygiene and nutrition in developed countries, and that readily available contraception and easy abortion mean that only babies who are wanted and can be supported economically are being born.

Both groups agree that more low-birth-weight and other problem babies survive today, in industrialized countries, because of the special, advanced pediatric care now available in hospitals. And both are aware that the continued high rate of maternal and infant deaths in the poor countries is due to two factors—malnourishment of mothers and infants and unsanitary conditions, particularly polluted water. In the most profoundly deprived countries (such as Bangladesh) a baby has only one chance in two of surviving past the age of five.

THE AMERICAN WAY OF BIRTH

Despite their complaints about their childbirth experiences, most women continue to be passive patients, which is "the American way." "The American public still expects the kind of medicine where the doctor is a savior," notes Israeli-born obstetrician Ilan Israeli, of the Mid-Island Hospital in Bethpage, New York. "The public demand here is for no pain, no real experience."

With all the goodwill in the world, American obstetricians accept the heavy responsibility of caring for patients who are dependent, ignorant, passive, and scared. They have chosen an area of medical practice that, perhaps more than any other, requires the full participation of a prepared and informed patient, yet once in it, everyone involved seems to pray only for uneventfulness. The possibilities for joy and pleasure in the childbirth experience—for the doctor as well as the patient—have been lost in the cold emphasis on technological improvement.

One evidence of how much our society reveres technology is that a doctor is more liable to be found guilty of malpractice today for *not* having used a new test or intervention than for intervening when anything goes wrong! If he listens to a baby's heartbeat with a stethoscope rather than an electronic fetal monitor (EFM), he is suspect. Only six years ago, it was the other way around, yet there is still no convincing proof that one method is better than the other, and using EFM carries certain risks and side effects.

Most of our innovations in aiding childbirth are technological rather than psychological. Doctors today can diagnose, medicate, even operate on a baby *in utero*, but have not stopped the rising number of premature births and undersized babies, which are so common among women who smoke and drink too much during pregnancy. Narcotics addiction in pregnant women is another serious problem caused by emotional and psychological factors. The number of addicted mothers has steadily increased. They give birth to babies who exhibit agonizing withdrawal symptoms. How many of these preemies could have been avoided with proper education and support?

Today more than 90 percent of mothers are drugged or anesthetized during childbirth. More than half our babies are "induced" to hurry up and come out. Forceps are still being used in more than half our hospital childbirths. The rate of abdominal births—known as cesarean sections— is up from 5 percent a decade ago to as high as 25 percent today in some parts of the country, and it is still rising.

Sophisticated medical equipment is used routinely in most births now or held close on hand "just in case." Patients are paying for expensive technological equipment and services whether they use them or not. In some hospitals, an anesthesiologist is assigned to every delivery, including natural childbirths, and the patient must pay his fee. Part of the reason that hospital costs are rising at such a phenomenal rate is that all these special services are very expensive.

A suburban East Coast uncomplicated delivery and three-day hospital stay can cost as much as $3000. How can young couples afford to have a baby? This may well be one of the reasons for the sharp rise in home births. People are beginning to object to the new technologies, not only because of their risks and side effects, but also because they cannot afford them.

Most babies are born in medical institutions whose rules were designed to isolate, protect, and treat sick people. Yet rigidity, impersonality, and enveloping regulation do not apply in the maternity situation. Many women are beginning to demand a more sympathetic setting.

Childbirth experts, too, are clamoring for a return to a more personalized hospital experience. "Much of the humanism in labor and delivery has been lost by the increased use of and dependence on technology," says Professor Jacqueline Rose Hott of the Adelphi School of Nursing in New York. "How do we know that these new technologies do not have harmful side effects?" asks natural childbirth teacher Jane Pittenger, of the Parent Effectiveness Training and Counseling Service of North Haven, Connecticut. "With every medical advance consumers need to be critical about safety factors."

The media are focusing attention on the relationship between the medical profession and the public it serves. Innovations are being extolled as "revolutionary breakthroughs," but the traditional relationship of authoritarian physician and passive patient is being questioned and criticized. Social psychologists have described this relationship as "learned helplessness." Learned helplessness is such a common disorder that people are unable to care for themselves in times of physical stress

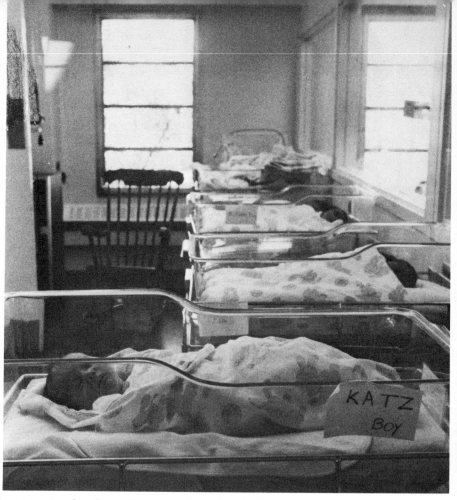

In America loneliness begins early when babies and mothers are routinely separated after birth. (Erika Stone)

because they believe their actions have little influence on the outcome of events. It is imperative to eradicate the traditional doctor-dependent relationship and initiate one of shared responsibility.

Some doctors and medical educators are waking up to the importance of this reeducation. "One of the important duties of a physician is to teach people how to care for themselves," says Dr. Catherine De Angelis, associate professor of Pediatrics and director of the Ambulatory Pediatric Service of the University of Wisconsin Medical School in Madison. "The majority of patients need preventive care as well as treatment of illnesses."

A few, like Dr. Lewis Mehl, director of the Berkeley Family Health Center and research director of the National Association of Parents and Professionals for Safe Alternatives in Childbirth (NAPSAC), would discard the old medical model altogether in favor of another concept: "A more useful concept is that of health-care provider, who works as an

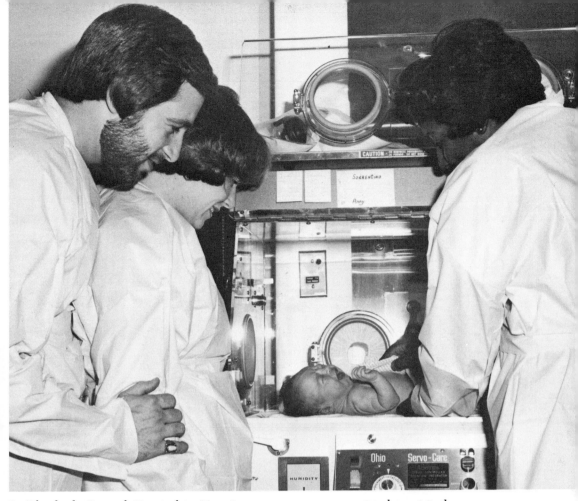

In Elizabeth General Hospital in New Jersey parents are permitted to visit the special-care unit and participate in the baby's care, an innovative feature comforting to parents. (Edward R. Bogard, Jr./Elizabeth General Hospital, Elizabeth, N.J.)

adviser rather than a prescriber. The client should be encouraged to look at his or her behavior and life-style and take responsibility for what effects these may be having on health problems."

Unless a pregnant woman has such an egalitarian relationship with her doctor—and most don't—she is likely to be made uncomfortable by such avant-garde ideas. And if she does decide to "see for herself," she will find the "facts" confusing, the research evidence conflicting, and the experts disagreeing about what is the best course for her to follow. No wonder young women, raised to be passively dependent on physicians, often ignorant about and fearful of childbirth, still refuse to take responsibility. It seems easier and more comforting to "trust in fate and the doctor."

Unfortunately, the consequences of such learned helplessness can reverberate for the rest of your life. Childbirth educators and psychologists report countless situations where the passive woman creates serious postpartum problems for herself and her family. Says Connecticut marriage counselor Jim Pittenger, of the Parent Effectiveness Training and Counseling Service of North Haven, Connecticut, "Often childbirth is a psychic trauma with the husband degraded in his wife's eyes. I believe the standard way of having babies puts marriages at risk."

In my own practice as a marriage counselor and psychotherapist, I have found surprisingly lively resentments from upsetting childbirth experiences. Clients relive with emotion those early days when they felt abandoned by their husbands, humiliated by their doctors, and overwhelmed by the unexpected responsibilities of motherhood. Some retaliated against their husbands by withholding sex. Others subtly discouraged intimacy between their husbands and their children. Relationships with their children suffered because childbirth and/or the first months afterward were so traumatic. Here's what one client confessed:

> "I always have rotten pregnancies. I feel sick the whole time, but I won't take anything because it could be bad for the baby. My childbirths were okay—I had spinals—but breast-feeding was hard for me. I never had enough milk, the babies cried, and even with my third baby my nipples hurt. But I breast-fed them all anyway, for three months, then I quit.
>
> "It was my husband's attitude that still bugs me the most. He was always in such a good mood about it all. With the first two, we lived in a garden project, and weekends, he'd be down playing ball with the other men on the street while I was upstairs with the baby. He always filled the living room with company, laughing and howling, while I was trying to breast-feed. I'd have to rock the babies to sleep for hours.
>
> "Later he made a lot of money. I was always close to the children, chauffering them to private school and ballet lessons. I really loved them when they were bigger. But I didn't love him. Sex was never very good, and it got worse with each pregnancy. He has these secretaries in the office and he travels a lot. But I don't care. I have the children."

THE SPECTER OF MALPRACTICE

Another result of traumatic childbirth is a mistrust of doctors. In first pregnancies, most women relate to their doctors with a childlike dependency and willing submissiveness. In fact, husbands sometimes resent the way their wives idealize their obstetricians and rave about them: "He's young and so easy to talk to. I don't have anyone else to talk to about the baby. He makes me feel so relaxed." When things go badly, positive feelings easily turn to sour resentment: "He was fine until the problems started." "He didn't want me to do any of the things I wanted to do." "I guess he's a good doctor, but he's in it for the money, right?" one disillusioned patient said. "After the delivery he yanked on the cord to make the afterbirth come, and then he left. I hemorrhaged on the table. Later, I found out what a bad thing that was to do," were the remarks of another.

The malpractice suit has become a standard recourse of the impotent, angry, and disappointed patient. These suits are rising at an alarming rate and have made the medical establishment—doctors and hospitals—overly cautious about returning to the simpler, less scientific procedures the public is now demanding. "It's the fear of malpractice suits that is preventing hospitals from being more flexible," says Dr. Robert Fitzgerald, former chief of the Long Island (New York) American Society for Psycho-Prophylaxis in Obstetrics doctors' group. Such humanistic procedures as allowing a mother to hold her baby on the recovery table or allowing her to be alone with her baby in a private room become more and more difficult to arrange, even though many doctors know how valuable such early intimacy can be in cementing the mother-child relationship.

The malpractice specter also has the effect of pressuring otherwise conservative doctors into using new technologies on *all* patients in order to have documented records of their procedures in case anything does go wrong. Even though a doctor is well aware of the discomforts and possible side effects of using an electronic fetal monitor, for example, he is also aware that he's more likely to be found guilty of malpractice if something goes wrong and he has not used the monitor than if he has. If he allows a breech baby to be delivered vaginally rather than by cesarean section, his procedure will be considered questionable in court, even though many breech babies can be born vaginally with no complications or danger to the mother or baby.

Thus the malpractice suit has created a vicious cycle in which physicians are guarded and defensive and patients are saddled with over-regulation and technology they neither need nor want. Pediatricians Seymour Goldblatt and Richard Todhunter of Alexandria, Virginia, claim, "Almost all physicians have become malpractice conscious. The best malpractice protection is a good doctor-patient relationship." But some mothers who have been enraged and disappointed by their obstetricians in childbirth find it impossible to establish a warm, trusting relationship with their pediatricians.

A COUNTERMOVEMENT

From experience, we know that both doctors and hospitals do respond to consumer pressure. Ten years ago, only 5 percent of fathers saw their children being born, and now an estimated 60 percent are allowed in delivery rooms.

In 1974, the International Childbirth Education Association (ICEA) conducted a nationwide survey of the status of family-centered childbirth throughout America. By then, 86 percent of fathers were allowed to stay with their wives during labor but not during delivery—and the figure may be close to 100 percent today. But in many places, that was the only change. Less than half our hospitals had childbirth preparation classes, rooming-in of mother and baby together, or any other family-centered feature. And the South lagged far behind the other regions of the country. Only about one-fourth of Southern hospitals had preparation classes, rooming-in, or allowed fathers in delivery rooms.

Family-centered childbirth in our hospitals still has a long way to go, but trends indicate that it is growing and becoming stronger. Many large medical centers are now offering maternity units with nurse-midwives in attendance and obstetrical backup, for example. In principle at least, the American College of Obstetricians and Gynecologists (ACOG) has been behind the family-centered hospital childbirth movement since 1975, when it said, "We recognize the concern of many that the events surrounding birth be an emotionally satisfying experience for the family." A 1977 ACOG survey of New York hospitals turned up this surprising finding: early discharge is now possible in more than 95 percent of hospitals. While the New York figure is undoubtedly higher than that for much of the rest of the country, it does indicate a growing acceptance by hospitals and doctors of parents' desires to be reunited at home as soon as it is medically safe. "The situation changes day by day," reports Doris Olson, president of ICEA. "What begins as an exception can soon become policy when the hospital sees that it works."

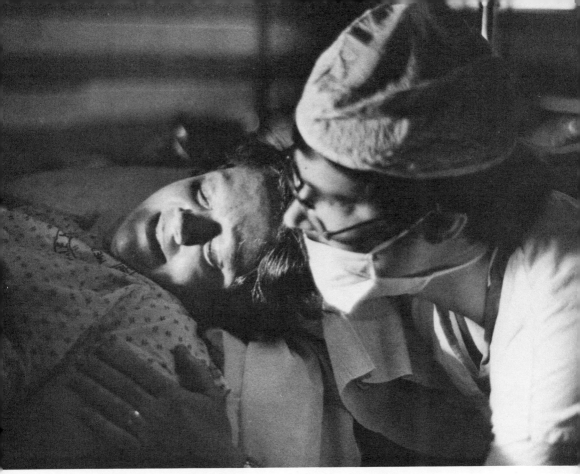

Emotional support is the "natural sedative" of childbirth. (Dr. David Kliot/Brookdale Hospital Medical Center)

"It requires effort on the doctor's part, but with that extra effort and a little more flexibility on the hospital's part, a lot can be accomplished," says Dr. Robert Fitzgerald. "Consumers are going to have to insist. Changes will continue to come about because of the consumer, with the help of the doctor."

More large hospitals are developing special units that have excellent provisions for family-centered childbirth. In the best of them, the mother comes to the hospital and labors and delivers in the same room, where she then stays with the baby until discharge. Her husband is present during labor and delivery and learns baby care alongside his wife before discharge. In some settings, other family members and friends can also be present, although this is still exceptional and experimental.

An important feature is the physical plant, now often very attractively furnished, more like a bedroom than a hospital room. It looks homey, but it is equipped even for surgery in some settings.

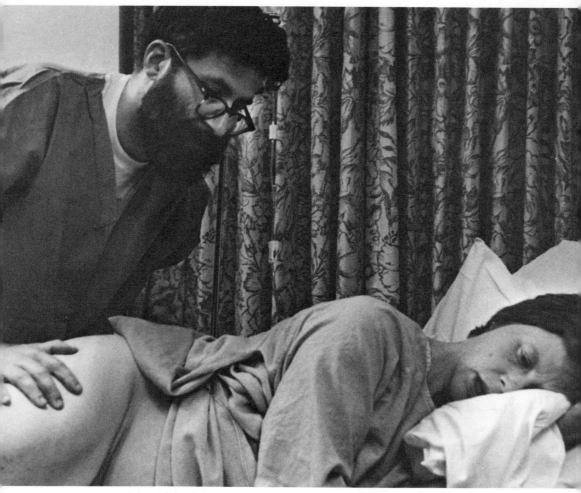

Back and leg massage is one more way the husband can help his wife relax during labor. (From the Parenting Pictures film: The Bonding Birth Experience, *Courter Films and Associates.)*

Elizabeth General Hospital in New Jersey has two types of rooms in its maternity unit. One, for early labor, is furnished like a living room. The other is for delivery and recovery. There is a community visiting room where relatives, friends, and children can come any time the mother is ready to see them. The nurseries to which the babies are removed for special care are thoughtfully located next to the special units. Most mothers and babies go home in twenty-four to forty-eight hours.

Breast-feeding also is increasing. A decade ago, only 5 percent of American women were able to breast-feed their babies for up to four months. Now that figure is 25 percent nationwide and as high as 45 percent on the West Coast. Although environmental pollutants in breast milk continue to be a problem, and the use of childbirth drugs has been shown to strongly affect a newborn infant's ability to suck on the breast, social attitudes toward breast-feeding are now so supportive that the upward trend seems to be continuing.

CHOOSING BETWEEN EXTREMES

In the next few years, couples will have to choose between extremes in hospital care. While homelike units are being established and special nurse-midwifery services are becoming more available, an opposite trend is also taking place. "Regionalization" is the name of a plan being implemented all over the country that involves the closing of smaller, less well equipped hospitals and the reliance on large medical centers that deliver two thousand or more babies a year and have technological equipment and special services for problem babies. In the regular maternity sections of these hospitals, routine technology like electronic fetal monitoring will be required.

It is ironic that the two trends are developing at the same time. Natural-childbirth advocates and technologists enthusiastically advocate their methods and have a great deal of evidence to back up the superiority of their approach. It will be up to you, to select the childbirth service that is best for you, just as knowledgeably as you buy any other product or service. It is therefore necessary to learn the advantages and disadvantages of each kind of childbirth. If a mother has a history of illness, or if her pregnancy is going poorly, her choice is clear. A large medical center, with the most advanced safeguards and equipment, is the safest place to be. In normal situations, however, when the mother is healthy and no problems are anticipated, the decision about birth setting can be based on the psychological needs of the mother. Even in such medical "gray areas" as twin deliveries and breech position, many mothers do better with natural childbirth in a homelike setting than they would in a regular hospital. Therefore, in some hospitals, nurse-midwives, using labor rooms for labor and delivery, will accept these cases for prepartum care and delivery, knowing there is an obstetrician close at hand if things go badly.

Studies have shown that women seem to select the right birth setting for themselves. Those who end up needing interventions usually have found their way to the larger medical centers. Those who do not are more likely to select natural-childbirth settings. Of course, many who select large hospitals have normal and uneventful births, and occasionally women have to be transferred to hospitals in the midst of home births.

If you would feel more comfortable and safe in a large, advanced medical setting, then that is the place for you. Many women have a great fear of childbirth, and the hospital atmosphere, which seems impersonal and cold to others, is reassuring to them.

Here is one woman's reason for choosing a traditional hospital: "I just want to have my baby the normal way, stay three days, and go home. . . . Everyone else is doing it this way. Why make waves?"

A second woman, who was prepared for natural childbirth in a local medical center, encountered considerable problems during delivery. Yet she found the setting supportive enough to offset any feelings of disappointment: "I had a fabulous pregnancy and trust in my doctors. I was two weeks overdue, and they suggested a stress test. The baby's heartbeat was weak, and they decided I needed a cesarean that day. I was disappointed that my husband couldn't be there, but they were all wonderful. The nurse stood there and talked to me the whole time— right from the test until after I had the baby. The doctors in the group all came around to see me every day. You know something—it was a great experience!"

Other women feel quite differently about hospitals. They are there for safety's sake, but would like to get out as soon as possible and be interfered with as little as necessary during their stay. These women found nurse-midwife natural-childbirth units in large hospitals for their deliveries. Here is what they told me:

"In my first delivery, I wanted my baby with me but I felt the nurses owned him. I actually cried when they handed the baby to me in the wheelchair as I was leaving. With the midwives, it was different. They were there only to help me. I felt I had control of my babies the whole time."

"They separated me from my husband for the prepping," another said of her hospital delivery. "I was pretty advanced in labor when I went in. Before he came back, I was in transition and losing control. A strange doctor came in and said, 'I have you down for epidural anesthesia.' I said it was a mistake, but then, a few minutes later, I said, 'Get that fellow back in here.' This second time [a twin delivery with nurse-midwives in attendance at a hospital] I felt that I had two people by my side ready to fight for me—my husband and the midwife. Three, actually. The second baby was breech, and they called an obstetrician in to stand by."

You, I—each of us is unique. Instinctively, you will find that you are attracted to certain settings. Visit a number of them, starting with your local hospital (the natural-childbirth teacher will let you tag along on a class tour). Visit the closest hospital that has a nurse-midwife unit, and meet the women there. There may be a hospital in your area with a birthing room—where you both labor and deliver your baby with your obstetrician in attendance—so check into that.

Look around for yourself. Like animals, we should spend time sniffing out the place where we will feel most comfortable giving birth!

Part Two:

MAPPING YOUR OWN ROUTE

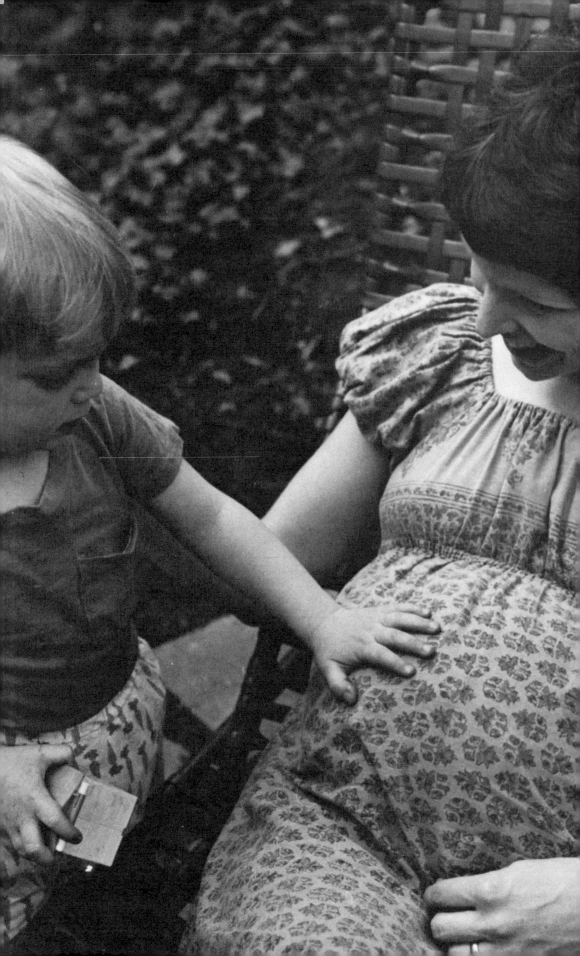

2

Becoming Body Centered

Luckily for the woman who is pregnant today, the "natural way"—eating nutritiously, avoiding body pollutants such as nicotine, caffeine, and alcohol, and exercising regularly—is becoming fashionable. Things were very different twenty years ago, when Princess Grace of Monaco announced she was planning to breast-feed her children and not worry about her spreading figure. "Now is *not* the time to care about my waistline," said Grace, quite unconventionally. But mistaken values still dominate, and "thin is beautiful" plagues even the pregnant woman. It is an attitude that is strongly embedded and difficult to shed during the childbearing years. A young woman's self-image depends a great deal on social expectations.

The available sound information about how to eat right and keep fit gets distorted by the omnipresent media image of the "ideal woman," the newest fad diets, and the constant selling of beauty gimmicks. American advertising emphasizes appearance and undermines the trend to be healthfully body centered. Because of the pressure of these superficial values, women respond (eagerly) to doctors who, although they should know better, insist on strict weight limitations in pregnancy.

Doctors are products of our culture, too, and some hold onto outdated ideas just because they're comfortable with them. The result of medical strictures against gaining weight is that in our rich nation we have far too many small, undernourished new babies and a rising prematurity rate. Also, pregnant women are continuing to smoke, without really knowing how dangerous it is, and this, too, contributes to the prematurity rate. Many women are malnourished, not because of poverty, but because of poor medical advice.

Doctors used to believe that diet restriction, leading to smaller babies, would make for easier deliveries. They used to think that low-salt diets would prevent toxemia of pregnancy (high blood pressure and pro-

Pregnancy can be a learning experience to bring you and your other children closer. (Erika Stone)

tein in the urine, sometimes leading to convulsions and coma, called eclampsia). Since the 1950s, they have been prescribing diuretics or "water pills" to more than half their patients to prevent edema (swelling because of fluid retention).

Now researchers know that a low-salt diet can *cause* toxemia (some believe toxemia actually is a disease of malnourishment), that more salt than usual is important in a pregnant woman's diet, that diuretics are dangerous, and that some swelling in childbirth is normal. The old regimen—strict weight control, low-salt diet, and diuretics—is being replaced by a new one—freer weight gain, salting food to taste, and *no* diuretics.

For psychological reasons, both doctors and mothers are having trouble giving up on the outdated, harmful methods. It is easier for women in our culture to respond to authoritarian doctors who manage them like bad children, scold them for gaining weight, and play on their anxiety about being fat than to grow up emotionally and become self-regulating.

Theoretically, pregnancy would seem the perfect time to learn about nutrition, to kick the junk-food-and-cigarettes-and-coffee habit. In actuality, it is the time when many women resist learning the facts and changing their eating habits. Why is this so?

Yesterday's teenager is expected to make a sudden and profound shift in her values and priorities as soon as she marries and becomes pregnant. She is no longer supposed to care only about her body's appearance. Now her body is a responsibility, a piece of equipment to be kept tooled and in top condition for the family's use. Only yesterday, she hadn't a care in the world beyond a pimple-free skin and a freshly blown hairdo. Today, she's holding down a job, keeping house, adjusting to marriage and a sexual relationship, and to top it all, she becomes pregnant. Now, suddenly, she's supposed to be constantly concerned about her health and her diet—all because of that baby inside her! No wonder many young pregnant women have second thoughts from time to time about motherhood.

There are also body changes to cope with. Being pregnant is exciting and usually a time of well-being, but for many women, it is also a time of anxiety and apprehension about whether they will measure up physically to the challenges: "Will I ever get my figure back?" "Will my husband lose interest in me sexually?" "Will the delivery go all right, or will I feel like a failure?" "Will I have the strength and patience to be a good mother?" One way to handle all these negative feelings and worries is to bury and deny them. What some frightened young women do is to ignore the reality of pregnancy by eating too little and following the same hectic schedule that wasn't healthy even before pregnancy. By faking it, wearing a veneer of casual unconcern, they try to smother their anxiety.

It is more common for young women to deal with their anxieties by putting themselves in their doctors' hands, washing their own of any responsibility. If the doctor orders strict weight control, low-salt diet, and diuretics, they follow blindly without asking why. They read his diet charts and try to eat the right foods, but since they must control their weight gain, they can't eat enough of the right foods to satisfy their healthy appetites. Good little girls, they suffer hunger pangs constantly (particularly in the last months when the baby's brain is developing) because they skip meals before weighing-in time at the doctor's office. Poor little girls, they are making themselves and their babies sick with all that unnecessary hunger!

Learn what your body needs to be strong during pregnancy. Take the responsibility, long denied, of caring for and about yourself. The groundwork for a trouble-free delivery, for successful breast-feeding, and for producing a healthy baby is laid during the nine months of happy, healthy eating.

NEW KNOWLEDGE ABOUT NUTRITION AND DRUGS

Doctors, like most of us, don't learn much about nutrition in school. But some outstanding doctors have contributed to our new knowledge about nutrition in childbirth. Dr. Agnes Higgins, of the Diet Dispensary in Montreal, Canada, has for thirty years been improving the diets of low-income mothers with remarkable results: their babies are bigger and healthier, and women with long histories of defective children or inability to carry to term have been helped to deliver normal children simply by eating nourishing foods. Here in the United States, Dr. Thomas Brewer has been working with our poor in the South and in California, and his results are just as outstanding. Brewer's research and activism—spreading the word about the importance of good diet in pregnancy—have been very influential in making doctors aware of the importance of

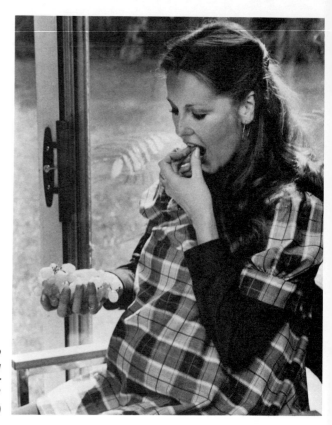

Dieting during pregnancy is no longer recommended by many nutritional experts. Satisfy your appetite with healthy foods!
(Erika Stone)

proper diet in pregnancy and in changing their medical management of pregnant women.

Dr. Higgins has strong evidence that spontaneous abortions, birth defects, and later disabilities are related to poor nutrition. Dr. Brewer believes he has demonstrated that there is a direct and causal relationship between malnutrition in pregnancy and the development of five common disorders: metabolic toxemia of pregnancy, abruption (premature detachment of the placenta, a major cause of fetal damage and maternal hemorrhage), severe infections, severe anemias, and a high percentage of low-birth-weight infants. His findings show that diuretics (pills to avoid water retention) have twenty-eight undesirable effects, including loss of appetite, stomach irritation, nausea, vomiting, cramps, diarrhea, muscle spasm, headache, and skin rash.

"EAT TO APPETITE, SALT TO TASTE"

In a recent interview, Dr. Brewer expressed his point of view:
"We have to get over our fear of weight gain and get into a fear of malnutrition, if we want healthy babies. In some poverty areas, up to 50 percent of babies are born sick, with sick mothers, and

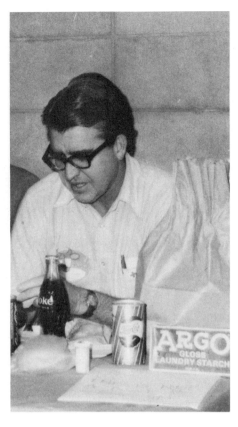

Dr. Thomas Brewer lectures widely with his "brown bag," which contains all the junk foods that lead to malnourishment in pregnancy. (Courtesy Dr. Tom Brewer)

this is as much nutritional in origin as it is due to poor birth practices. Nonwhites have twice the infant mortality of whites, and different parts of the country have different rates. . . . Malnutrition is leading to toxemia and eclampsia, and middle-class women are dying of malnutrition because of poor diet practices recommended by their doctors. The lowest infant mortality in America is in the Chinese and Japanese communities, which are 'eat for two' cultures, with traditional patterns of adequate, balanced diets.

"But doctors still aren't being taught applied nutrition in medical school. Where is the research that proves salt, weight restriction, and diuretics are valuable? We do know now that the baby is not a complete parasite, as we used to think, feeding off the mother, but must be fed well *in utero*. There is absolutely no rational basis for rigid weight control. Research studies done by the National Institutes of Health show that the lowest incidence of mental and motor abnormalities occur in pregnancies with high weight gain, with babies of higher weight. Insufficient salt leads to leg cramps and fatigue, and Margaret Robinson in London reported that low-salt diets resulted in twice as many babies dying and two and a half times more mothers getting toxemia.

For over a decade in the United States, two million women used diuretics each year. It is a big business for the drug industry. But diuretics can cause minimal brain dysfunction and learning disabilities in children.

"A woman should not restrict her weight gain but put all her emphasis on correct eating habits. She must never starve herself in the last months, when the baby's brain is developing. Long labors are directly related to the way the uterus grows in pregnancy, and that relates to a mother's nutrition. There is plenty of research evidence that one quart of milk a day, two eggs, meat and fish, vegetables, fruits, and whole grains—eighty to one hundred grams of protein a day—and the avoidance of junk foods are necessary to keep the developing baby and mother healthy. Even figure-conscious women will respond to this advice to eat a high-quality diet. We must stop looking at food as a recreation!

"Because we are a pill-popping culture, some middle-class women take a lot of vitamins and are unaware that they still may be malnourished. The idea of just eating a good diet is too simple in our drug-oriented culture. Vitamins are not a substitute for good food; they simply replace the nutrients removed by processing. Don't get false security from vitamin supplements."

Here is the diet that Dr. Brewer has been recommending for twelve years at the Contra Costa County, California, Prenatal Clinic Nutrition Education Project.

A Nutritious Diet for Pregnancy

When you are pregnant, you need more of good-quality foods than when you are not pregnant. To meet your own needs and those of your developing baby, you must have, *every day*, at least:

1. One quart (4 glasses) of milk—any kind: whole milk, low-fat, skim, powdered skim, or buttermilk. If you do not like milk, you can substitute one cup of yogurt for each cup of milk.
2. Two eggs.
3. Two servings of fish, shellfish, chicken or turkey, lean beef, veal, lamb, pork, liver, or kidney.

Alternative combinations include:
Rice with: beans, cheese, sesame, milk.

Cornmeal with: beans, cheese, tofu, milk.
Beans with: rice, bulgar, cornmeal, wheat noodles, sesame seeds, milk.
Peanuts with: sunflower seeds, milk.
Whole-wheat bread or noodles with: beans, cheese, peanut butter, milk, tofu.

For each serving of meat, you may substitute these quantities of cheese:

Brick—4 oz.	Longhorn—3 oz.
Camembert—6 oz.	Muenster—4 oz.
Cheddar—3 oz.	Monterey Jack—4 oz.
Cottage—6 oz.	Swiss—4 oz.

4. Two servings of fresh, green leafy vegetables: mustard, beet, collard, dandelion, or turnip greens, spinach, lettuce, cabbage, broccoli, kale, Swiss chard.
5. Five servings of whole-grain breads, rolls, cereals, or pancakes: wheatena, 100 percent bran flakes, granola, shredded wheat, wheat germ, oatmeal, buckweat or whole-wheat pancakes, corn bread, corn tortillas, corn or bran or whole-wheat muffins, waffles, brown rice.
6. Two choices from: a whole potato (any style), large green pepper, grapefruit, lemon, lime, orange, papaya, tomato (one piece of fruit or one large glass of juice).
7. Three pats of margarine (Vitamin A-enriched) or butter.

Also include in your diet:

8. A yellow- or orange-colored vegetable or fruit five times a week.
9. Liver once a week.
10. Table salt: SALT YOUR FOOD TO TASTE.
11. Water: Drink to thirst.

It is not healthy for you and your unborn baby to go even twenty-four hours without good food!

SOME SURPRISING FACTS

• While some important things, like protein, must be fed directly to the baby, he is parasitic in some ways. Calcium *is* drawn from the mother's body. Plenty of milk, milk products, even bone-meal supplements, are a good idea to prevent tooth loss and decay.

- Women on reducing diets have babies who are more vulnerable to illness.
- America's prematurity rate is rising, and a premature baby is at thirty times the risk of a normal-weight baby.
- The weight gain left after pregnancy may be nature's way of preparing for breast-feeding, which uses up to one thousand calories a day.

Studies show that mothers who drink excessively or smoke excessively are more apt to have low-birth-weight and premature babies. Many doctors agree that in addition to poor nutrition, smoking is a major reason for the small size of babies. A recent bulletin issued by the American College of Obstetricians and Gynecologists reports that pregnant mothers who smoke regularly run twice the risk of non-smokers of delivering a low-birth-weight infant. While a causal relationship between smoking and poor fetal growth has been acknowledged since the early 1970s, a strong dose relation is now evident. The negative effects of smoking on fetal growth have been shown to be directly proportional to the number of cigarettes smoked each day. If a mother stops smoking by the fourth month of pregnancy, however, her risk of delivering a low-birth-weight infant can be reduced to that of a non-smoker.

A "fetal alcoholism syndrome"—growth deficiences, mental abnormalities, and motor dysfunction—has been related to moderate and heavy alcohol consumption during pregnancy. According to Dr. Kenneth Warren of the National Institute on Alcohol Abuse and Alcoholism, a pregnant woman should not have more than one to two drinks a day (one drink equals one-half ounce of liquor). Mothers who take from three to five drinks a day run a great risk of causing a partial fetal alcohol syndrome, which results in learning disabilities and slower growth of the entire body. More than six drinks a day produces complete fetal alcohol syndrome with resulting mental retardation and the inability to progress into normal puberty. Ten percent of pregnant mothers in America today suffer fetal alcohol syndrome to some extent.

- "After feeling perfectly well on a good diet, after eighteen days on a 'zero protein' diet a patient went into toxemia."—Brewer.
- "Potato chips cost more than steak. Milk is cheaper and healthier than steak.'—Brewer.

COMMUNICATE EARLY WITH YOUR DOCTOR

Dr. Brewer feels that a weight gain of thirty-five to forty-five pounds is quite all right during pregnancy. "Studies show that weight gain or loss is irrelevant to whether a baby is normal. I don't discuss weight with the mother, I just ask her what she's eating."

Most American doctors do still follow weight guidelines, although they are more flexible than in past years. It is very important to find a doctor who is up to date on nutrition and permissive about weight gain. It is much harder to fight about this issue later when you are in the middle of pregnancy and he wants you to diet or take diuretics. Dieting is *harmful* in pregnancy. If your doctor insists, remember *you* are the one who will take the consequences. You are entitled to make your own decision about weight gain. 2072691

Of course, a discussion with the doctor will be easier now that you have some of the facts at your fingertips. If you want more information, write to SPUN (The Society for the Protection of the Unborn through Nutrition), Suite 603, 17 West Wabash Avenue, Chicago, Illinois 60602. Dr. Brewer and associates started this organization a few years ago to collect case histories, conduct research, prepare litigation, influence medical education and legislation, and give free information to the public. Dr. Brewer told me that they recently won their first case for nutritional malpractice.

SPUN can supply case histories of every sort: women who carried to term and had healthy children after repeated miscarriages; improved birth outcomes for teenage mothers who learned to eat properly; babies born with defects or stillborn because of poor nutritional advice or drugs prescribed by their doctors.

Research about over-the-counter drugs indicates that the safest course is to avoid *all* drugs and additives during pregnancy. A drug may be safe in itself, but harmful to the fetus in combination with another equally innocent drug. Avoid: aspirin, sedatives, antihistamines, barbiturates, diuretics, hormones, appetite suppressants, antacids, cough medicines, and tranquilizers. Jaundice, bleeding, even cleft palate in babies are thought to be associated with these frequently prescribed and freely available drugs.

SHOPPING WITHIN THE SYSTEM

It may be easier to find fresh, wholesome, and nutritious foods in expensive specialty shops, but it is also possible to eat well if you shop at your neighborhood supermarket. By purchasing carefully and knowledgeably, checking for freshness, and studying labels and codes, you can make sure that the food you eat is wholesome and contains a minimum of additives. Here are some guidelines to help you:

1. Wherever possible, buy whole grains and natural foods rather than processed and enriched products.
2. Don't assume that a product contains anything nutritious unless it is listed in the ingredients.
3. Many products, by law, list ingredients in descending order of predominance, but not all foods are required to do so. Many staples— including breads, canned fruits, juices, and vegetables—are simply supposed to maintain mandatory standards.
4. Read labels. The nutritional information will help you determine in which category of your recommended diet the food belongs.
5. Some products are given a grade, which means they meet certain government specifications.
6. Although codes differ from place to place, some cities and states have laws calling for clear marking of certain perishables. Always check perishables to find the freshest product available. Ask the store manager to explain the code if you don't understand it.
7. In most cases, nationally distributed items show the date of manufacture.
8. Baked goods are supposed to be kept on the shelf for only forty-eight hours before being marked down.
9. Use your eye to determine freshness of fruits and vegetables.
10. Meats are supposed to be marked with the day and time of cutting. Precooked meats should be consumed within days of purchase.
11. Frozen products may have been on the supermarket shelf for months, so don't keep them too long after purchase. Always check for signs of improper freezing, like softness, ice crystals, or package discoloration.
12. In some cities, dairy products must be marked with a date after which they cannot be sold. Check the container.

13. Eggs should be kept refrigerated in the supermarket and marked with a "pull date." Check this with the store manager.

Many women first become involved with diet and nutrition in pregnancy. The care with which they shop in order to protect the health of the unborn baby is excellent training for feeding the family in the years ahead.

EXERCISE, BUT TAKE IT EASY

Women respond enthusiastically to exercise before, during, and after pregnancy and childbirth. We are all figure-conscious, and while we are waiting for the baby to be born, many of us have extra time on our hands, and just enough apprehension and edginess so that a physical workout can be tension-relieving. Exercise in pregnancy can help you carry the baby more comfortably, and is relaxing and strengthening. Staying in touch with your body, learning what it can and cannot do, is good insurance that you will be able to handle the physical stresses to come.

Walking, swimming, dancing are all excellent—if they're your usual and favorite exercises. Some women play tennis through a large part of their pregnancy. (Check with your doctor if you want to continue this sport.)

During pregnancy, most women feel at their peak of energy and well-being. It is the one time of your life when you don't have to worry about keeping your stomach tucked in! The emphasis, physically as well as psychologically, should be on carrying the baby gracefully and comfortably. Enjoy your spreading silhouette instead of worrying about how to restore your figure afterward.

Some childbirth teachers are including fitness exercises along with breathing drills and relaxation exercises. Others prefer dance movement to help women learn to balance their increasing weight. All will tell you it is not muscle development but your state of mind and your feelings about your body that will help you through a normal labor and delivery. Mechanical control and muscular development can be overdone. Some women work too hard at exercise as a way of overcoming apprehension about the coming childbirth.

One advantage of a prepartum exercise class is that the teacher can design an individual program for you based on your body's needs. But it

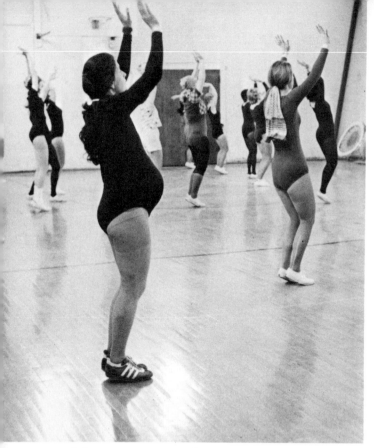

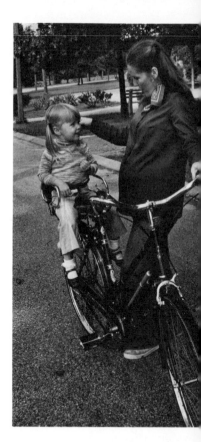

Top left: At a YWCA aerobic dance class a pregnant woman takes class through to the end of her term.(Alison Ehrlich Wachstein, from Pregnant Moments, Morgan & Morgan, *1978)*

Top right: Deciding with your doctor how much you can do without undue stress is important.(Erika Stone)

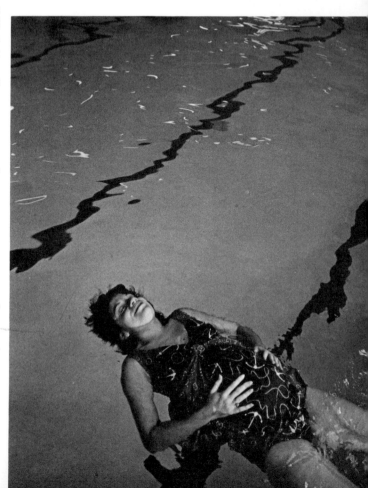

Bottom right: Body-toning exercises like walking and swimming are good for every healthy pregnant woman. (Alison Ehrlich Wachstein, from Pregnant Moments, Morgan & Morgan, *1978)*

is quite all right to do exercises on your own at home, designing a schedule to suit yourself. It is also fine to omit formal exercises entirely so long as you follow your usual active recreations during pregnancy. Just take care to avoid strain and exhaustion. Keep in mind that staying fit and having fun are equally important.

Prepartum Fitness Exercises

These exercises, the pelvic floor exercises, the postpartum exercises, and the cesarean preparation and rehabilitation exercises, are reprinted with the permission of Marilyn Freedman, president of the Long Island ASPO, childbirth education teacher in the Lamaze method, and professional physiotherapist. She urges that you check with your doctor before undertaking them, since some doctors feel that no exercise program is safe in the first three months of pregnancy, when miscarriages are possible.

All exercises are to be done on a firm surface, as smoothly and rhythmically as possible, without any discomfort or strain. Stop *before* becoming fatigued. Unless otherwise indicated, begin with 5 repeats of an exercise, slowly increasing by 1 repeat a day until you are doing 10 to 15. Intersperse stomach, leg, and back exercises.

Exercise 1. To improve circulation, prevent or ease swollen feet and legs and varicose veins.
Position: Lie with pillow under head and legs elevated and fully supported at about 45 degrees (on inverted chair).
(a) Point knees to ceiling, bend and straighten feet, all the way up and down at ankle, 30 times.
(b) Part legs slightly, rotate feet in as large a circle as possible, with legs still relaxed and supported, working at the ankle only, 15 times in each direction.
(c) Press thighs together, push knees down, contract buttocks tightly. Hold 5 seconds, then release.
Exercise 2. Abdominal muscle exercise to strengthen stomach muscles.
Position: Lie flat with knees bent up and feet flat on floor.
(a) Pelvic tilt (rocking the baby)—Place one hand in the hollow of

your back, the other on your hipbone. Slowly tighten stomach and buttocks. As you flatten back against your hand, feel the hipbone move backward and buttocks lift slightly. Breathe out as you tighten muscles, breathe in as you release. Do *not* arch back upward. Maintain contraction 4–5 seconds, release slowly.

Progression: Do the same exercise with legs extended.

(b) Stretch hands out in front of you, reach toward knees, pelvic tilt. Blow out and slowly arch up, tucking your chin in first, coming up vertebra by vertebra as you lift head and shoulders off the ground. Go as far as you are comfortable going, not more than 45 degrees. Blow out as you come up and breathe in as you uncurl.

Note: If your abdominal muscles bulge in a point as you come up, do the exercises anyway, but hold the two sides of the abdominal muscles together because it means they have split. (A common non-serious occurrence.)

(c) Pelvic tilt and curl up, vertebra by vertebra, reaching out over left knee with your hands, looking behind you to the left. Breathe in, then curl down slowly. Repeat on right side.

(d) Draw in abdominal muscles as you blow out. Hold 5 seconds and release slowly.

Exercise 3. Inner thigh stretching, to make the position of delivery easier.

Position: Sit, heels together and close to your crotch.

(a) Place right hand on feet and left hand under knee.

(b) Give counterpressure with left hand under left knee, push knee down to the floor, using your muscles against the pressure of your hand.

(c) Relax and repeat 5 times.

(d) Repeat procedure, using right hand and right knee.

Exercise 4. To prevent back injuries by strengthening spinal muscles and stabilizing spine.

Position: Kneel on all fours.

(a) Lift right arm and left leg to make a straight line with back. Do *not* allow back to arch or hollow. Hold 5 seconds and lower gently.

(b) Lift left arm and right leg, hold 5 seconds, and lower gently. Then—do **pelvic rock** to strengthen abdominal muscles, relieve backache and constipation. Slowly pull buttocks in (like a dog with a tail between its legs); at the same time, tighten abdominal muscles and blow out. Hold 5 seconds, then relax.

Exercise 5. To help support heavier breasts by strengthening the underlying pectoral muscles.
Position: Sit in tailor position, legs crossed.
(a) Grip your forearms firmly just above the wrists, right hand on left wrist, and vice versa.
(b) Raise elbows to shoulder level.
(c) Apply pressure through your hands toward your elbows, feeling the tightening in the muscles under your breast.
(d) Relax.

Exercise 6. Foot Exercises. To strengthen foot muscles and prevent flattened arches and poor posture.
Position: Sit with soles of feet flat on floor.
(a) Push your toes down on the floor, keeping them straight and making an arch underneath them. Do *not* curl toes. Relax.
(b) Spread toes as far apart as you can. Then bring them together.
Progression: Do the same exercises standing.

Exercise 7.—Pelvic tilt. To help maintain good muscle tone and posture.
Position: Stand, chin tucked in and head high.
Tip the baby back in its cradle by tightening the abdominal muscles and tucking your buttocks between your legs. Blow out as you do this, then relax.

Exercise 8.—Hip hiking (duck walk). To strengthen abdominal muscles.
Position: Stand.
(a) While standing on left leg, hitch right leg up into waist, keeping leg straight. Relax. Repeat with left leg.

Exercise 9.—Half-squats. To strengthen thigh muscles, for more efficient lifting.
Position: Stand on nonslippery floor, holding on to something heavy and solid.
(a) Place right foot in front of left.
(b) Slowly lower left knee to the floor, keeping head up and bottom tucked under.
(c) Stand upright slowly.
(d) Repeat with opposite leg, lowering right knee to ground.

There is one set of exercises developed by physiotherapists in childbirth education, called pelvic floor exercises, sexercises, or Kegel Exercises (named for Dr. Arnold Kegel of the University of California in Los Angeles, who was among the first physicians to recognize their importance). These are recommended to all as an important preparation for labor and delivery and for proper restoration of the pelvic floor muscles after childbirth. During pregnancy, there is a great deal of pressure on the pelvic floor muscles. The stronger they are, the better will be the support for your uterus and other pelvic organs during pregnancy, and the better you will know how to relax them during childbirth. By training these muscles now, you will be better able to reeducate them afterward. A healthy, exercised muscle is restored much sooner than a neglected one.

These exercises are recommended for *all* women, not just those of childbearing age. In fact, they are even more essential as a woman gets older. Fifty percent of American women suffer from weakness of the pelvic floor, which throughout life is stressed by such ordinary activities as laughing, coughing, sneezing, lifting, straining, pushing during the second stage of labor, and waste elimination. Pregnancy, because of the enlarging uterus, causes increasing and long-standing pressure on the pelvic floor.

A strong pelvic floor can withstand the pressures that occur in normal life, particularly childbirth, and can provide sphincter control of the perineal openings—the urethra, vagina, and anus. Symptoms of a weak pelvic floor range from vague aches and fatigue all the way to urinary incontinence and leakage and prolapse of the uterus. Sometimes the uterus actually bulges through the vaginal outlet and requires surgery for correction.

These exercises should begin before pregnancy, continue postpartum, and then become part of a woman's daily fitness program for the rest of her life. They are particularly helpful in healing after an episiotomy and in restoring sexual functioning after childbirth.

Pelvic Floor Exercises (Sexercises)

NOTE: These exercises are for the two main groups of muscles forming a figure 8 surrounding the urethra and vagina and the anus. All the muscles insert into the perineal body, a fibrous circle of tissue between the vagina and anus. It is impossible to move one group of muscles without the other, but trying will give you a good feeling of the difference between them. The muscles are very thin and tire easily. Do only five good contractions at a time, holding for only five seconds before releasing.

Exercise 1. To isolate and contract the pelvic floor muscles.

Position: Lie down, one pillow under head and one under knees.

(a) Cross one leg over the other. Squeeze legs tightly together, tighten buttock muscles, and pull up as if you need to urinate but must wait. This is only to help you locate the muscles. In other exercises, you do not contract abdominal or buttock muscles, but *isolate* pelvic floor muscles.

(b) Lie down, legs released and not crossed. Tighten only pelvic floor muscles, all the way up into the vagina.

(c) Isolate the contraction to just the urethra and vagina (a tiny movement).

(d) Isolate the contraction to just around the anus (a larger movement).

Note: A fingertip placed at the lips of the vagina or at the opening of the anus will enable you to feel the difference in these contractions.

(e) Elevator exercise: Imagine the pelvic floor as an elevator. With each stop, pull the floor up a little more. Do not let go between stops. Then descend floors, letting the contraction go one stop at a time. In the basement (complete relaxation), you will be able to feel the muscles bulging slightly downward, like a miniature hammock. Go even one stop or floor lower than that (by pushing down)—to the subbasement. The vaginal lips will open slightly, and you will have to hold your breath or blow out slightly to feel this. (This is the position your pelvic floor should be in when you are being examined internally or while the baby is being born.)

NOTE: Always end this exercise by going back up to the first floor again. A certain amount of tone in the pelvic floor muscles should be maintained during the day. The pelvic floor has a "correct posture."

Progression: Do exercise with legs spread wide apart.
Do exercise sitting, with legs relaxed and apart.
Do exercise standing.

Exercise 2. Bathroom exercises. (Yes, you do these in the bathroom!)

(a) Start and stop the flow of urine *a few times*. (Some urologists feel that overdoing this exercise may lead to incomplete emptying of the bladder, causing a urinary infection. So don't do the exercise more than a few times every few days. You also can avoid incomplete emptying by taking the pelvic floor to the "subbasement.")

(b) Feel the difference in sensations between consciously passing urine and letting it pass out passively.

(c) Pass a stool, first pushing and then passively. Particularly during pregnancy, pass stool passively. Help by blowing air out of your mouth through pursed lips. This will avoid building up too much pressure and decrease the possibility of hemorrhoids.

Exercise 3. Lovemaking exercise.

During intercourse, grip the penis with your vaginal muscles. This usually is extremely pleasant for the male. Your muscles will tire easily at first but consistent exercise strengthens them and improves sexual pleasure, both during pregnancy and for future lovemaking, for you and your mate. Don't overdo; these muscles build up over a period of months.

Called sexercises, all these are used to help preorgastic women in sex therapy.

From a psychological point of view, I recommend that you attend a class for exercise after the baby comes. A regular commitment to going out will help restore your perspective on life. It is a good way of meeting other women to socialize with during baby-carriage days. Before you go to a class, the graded exercises below will begin to restore prepregnancy fitness.

Postpartum Exercises

Once a day, lie on your stomach, with pillows under your abdomen, hips, and head to avoid pressure on milk-filled breasts. Remain in this position for at least 20 minutes. This helps the uterus move forward into a good position.

Do the following exercises in the hospital and on your return home, slowly and in sustained movements. Exercise for short periods (5 minutes) a number of times a day. Each day add new exercises to the ones that are indicated for the days before. Some of these exercises are taken from the prepartum fitness and pelvic floor exercises outlined on page 43.

Day One

Diaphragmatic breathing. Breathe in deeply through your nose, feeling your waistline expand. Blow out through your mouth, pulling in abdominal muscles.

Sexercises (p. 43). Do a different one at each session.

Foot movements (For circulation). Circle foot, pump foot, lying or sitting down.

Day Two

Pelvic rock. (p. 40)

Head and shoulder raising. (2(b), Prepartum Fitness Exercises)

Pelvic floor exercises and Pelvic rocking in standing position.

Day Three

Pelvic swinging.

Position: Lie, knees up, feet flat on bed.

Keep knees tightly together and drop legs to one side. Lift slowly, drop legs to other side. Begin by dropping legs only until your stitches begin to hurt. Eventually you will be able to get all the way down.

Foot exercises. (p. 41)

Day Four

Abdominal muscle exercise. See Exercise 2(b) in Prepartum Fitness Exercises.

Hold sides of abdominal muscles together if split.

Bridging.

Position: Lie down, knees bent, feet flat on bed.

Lift buttocks into the air.

Lower-back strengthener.

Position: Lie on stomach, pillow under hips, arms resting along sides. Lift head and shoulders 5 times.

Day Five

Hip hiking. See Exercise 8 in Prepartum Fitness Exercises.

Abdominal muscles. See Exercise 2(c) in Prepartum Fitness Exercises.

Note: Do only if muscles are *not* split.

Breast muscle exercise. See Exercise 5 in Prepartum Fitness Exercises.

You can begin this if your milk supply is established and not excessive. If you're bottle-feeding, wait until all traces of milk have disappeared before starting. Exercise is useful for *building up* milk supply.

Continue exercises, increasing the number of times as you feel stronger. Here are some additional exercises, once you feel up to them:

1. This progression for the abdominal exercises given below involves increasing resistance.

    (a) Lie down, hands across chest. Roll body up slowly, never jerk. When this is easy, proceed to (b).

    (b) Place hands behind neck, with elbows out to sides, roll up and down as in (a).

2. Keeping back perfectly straight, pelvic tilt and do a half-squat (*never* a full squat).

3. Once postpartum discharge (lochia) has stopped, pelvic tilt on all fours.

4. Lift one arm and the other leg. This strengthens your back.

These exercises will get you back in shape in the first six weeks and prepare you for an exercise class, which most doctors recommend you do *not* start until after your six-week checkup.

3
Your First Choice:

Managed or
Natural Childbirth

Essentially, there are two ways to go in childbirth—medical management or the natural route. For most women, prepartum care and delivery are with an obstetrician. So what then are the differences between these two alternatives?

One is your perception and your doctor's perception of what childbirth is. Two is your perception and your doctor's perception of what your relationship to one another should be during your entire childbirth experience.

How do *you* see childbirth? Do you think of it as normal and natural, or as stressful, painful, and potentially dangerous? You will find that experts hold both points of view, and have impressive arguments and studies to back up their views.

Here are the opinions of some leading childbirth educators who teach us that for most women a natural, unmanaged childbirth, without intervention and drugs, is not only possible but necessary for a good outcome for both mother and baby:

"Childbirth is not an illness, but work for which the body is efficiently and exquisitely constructed. It should be truly a happy event, taking place in an atmosphere of tranquility and loving care. Teams of skilled nurses, batteries of sterile instruments, rows of antiseptically clean and shining delivery rooms and spotless nurseries shielded by glass plate cannot ensure that this atmosphere is created."—Sheila Kitzinger, The Natural Childbirth Trust, London, England.

"Childbirth is a transcendental experience. It is one of life's great adventures. For some of us, the present American way of birth is totally destructive to some aspect of our existence."—Lester Hazell, Center for Special Problems in San Francisco.

It is their view that the traditional American way of having babies—in the hospital, with frequent interventions into what is an essentially normal process—creates many of the problems American women experience in childbirth:

"Obviously, there will always be medical indications that dictate the use of various obstetrical procedures, but to apply these practices routinely to the vast majority of mothers who are capable of giving birth without complication is to create added stress. . . . Most of the world's mothers receive little or no drugs during pregnancy, labor, and birth. Constant emotional support greatly improves a mother's tolerance of discomfort. In American labor rooms, drugs rather than skillful emotional support are employed."—Doris Haire, Foundation for Maternal and Child Health and Family Planning.

Some physicians hold that exact view. They agree with Dr. Roberto Caldeyro-Barcia, president of the International Association of Obstetrics and Gynecologists, who says, "Only act when there is a deviation from normality. Otherwise do not intervene." But many more believe routine safeguards are necessary for all women, since it is impossible, in their view, to predict which childbirths will be hazardous. Here is a sampling of the views of doctors who advocate carefully monitored and managed hospital childbirths:

"You never know at the beginning of a labor what might be needed. Ten percent of deliveries get into trouble, deliveries where you cannot anticipate trouble. Labor is natural, but it is a hazardous process."—Dr. Stanley James, professor of Pediatrics, Obstetrics, and Gynecology, Columbia University College of Physicians and Surgeons, New York.

Dr. Richard H. Aubry, who is chairman of the American College of Obstetricians and Gynecologists in New York State, is also very concerned about the trend toward viewing childbirth as normal and unhazardous. He says, "The perinatal period—the last five months of pregnancy and the first month of newborn life—still represents the single riskiest time of an individual's life until the ills of old age begin to take their toll."

Some natural-childbirth doctors caution against overstated claims of "painless childbirth." Dr. Benjamin Segal, who was a founding member of the American Society for Psycho-Prophylaxis in Obstetrics (ASPO), the organization that has done the most to promote natural childbirth in the United States, put it very well: "Labor can be perceived in degrees, varying from simple awareness to intense pain. . . . The patient's attitudes toward her pregnancy, her social and medical history, her relationship with her husband, the unborn child, and the physician all affect her responses."

And Dr. Mieczyslaw Finster, professor of Anesthesiology at Columbia University College of Physicians and Surgeons, has this view: "It is not only a matter of preparation and personality. It is a matter of the type and direction of labor whether a mother will be able to withstand the pain."

These are the assessments of qualified experts. In the end, it is your own perception of childbirth that will determine which arguments are more persuasive. You must also assess your feelings about the doctor-patient relationship. Natural-childbirth advocates feel that a mother should never abdicate responsibility for herself. She should be educated to make informed choices and to share decision making with the doctor: "Unless you take the time to learn about labor from an objective standpoint, to learn about what your community offers by way of support for you, and most important, take the time to really know yourself and what your emotions are, then you truly have no choice," says Lester Hazell.

Medical sociologist Doris Haire adds this important point: "You must demand that obstetricians prove to you their method is better."

Only natural-childbirth doctors, who want their patients to be "awake and aware," share this point of view. The medical-management opinion is that what is of primary importance is the mother's confidence in her doctor, which enables her to place full responsibility for the outcome in his hands.

"In the last twenty years, obstetrics has become a science, and women are rejecting it," says Dr. Finster. "The movement to humanize childbirth in a hospital setting is a healthy one," says Dr. James. "However, because of the potential dangers to the infant, there is a serious question as to whether the mother has a right to reject the benefits of modern obstetric care. While the mother has rights, so has the baby if he is to survive labor and delivery intact."

Deciding who holds the final responsibility is difficult. It requires undertaking a thorough, self-education about childbirth and the options for delivery, selecting a doctor as much on the basis of your personal response to him and your ability to communicate with him easily as on his credentials and reputation. Most importantly, it requires a willingness to evaluate your emotional needs, temperament, and philosophy.

I have designed the following questionnaire to help you decide between medically managed and natural childbirth.

GETTING IN TOUCH WITH YOUR FEELINGS

Be honest in your answers. It is okay to discuss the issues with your husband or other people involved with your childbirth, but is is *your* feelings that matter most.

1. What would be your ideal childbirth experience? Would you want to be asleep or awake during delivery? Why? At home or in the hospital? Why? Who would be there?

2. Are you afraid of drug-free childbirth? Why? Of drugs and anesthesia? Why? What would help you overcome these fears?

3. Do hospitals frighten or reassure you? Describe the best possible hospital experience for you. Is the hospital you prefer small and private or a large training hospital with every facility? Are you alone in the room or with other women? Is the baby there? Is your husband there? Do you have visitors? Who comes?

4. Are you interested in a home birth? Why? Would you rather be assisted by a doctor or a midwife? Why?

5. How important is it to you as a couple to share the birth experience? (This is an important question. Some husbands do not want to be present, or are halfhearted about it. Some wives would rather not have their husbands there, even though it is unfashionable to admit this. You must both be honest in your answers.) If you aren't sure how you feel, this is an area you can discuss and explore by seeing films and attending classes together.

6. How much time and effort are you willing to invest in motherhood? Full time? For how long? Do you want to continue a social life? Work? (Your decision about breast-feeding, discussed later, is at issue here. For most women, breast-feeding means full-time motherhood in the first months.)

On the basis of this first assessment, you should have a clearer idea than before of your feelings. You may be leaning more in the direction of medical management than you had suspected. As Lester Hazell points out, "We bring our entire history into labor, our whole personality." If you think you would feel safer in a hospital, under traditional medical management, keep these feelings in mind as you read the next chapter about the hospital experience and about drugs and some of the newer interventions. Then you can come to a final decision based on knowledge, not just feelings.

Similarly, if you incline toward natural childbirth, or home birth, read the relevant chapters carefully. Whether they support your feelings or change them, when you make your final choice, you will know it is based on knowledge, not blind faith.

Childbirth is a learning experience. The setting and method you choose for a first childbirth may change in subsequent ones. Whatever the outcome, you are making the best choice you can. There is nothing to feel guilty about.

4

Medically Managed and Monitored Childbirth

Until World War II, half of America's babies were born at home. Many mothers had no prenatal care. Our maternal mortality was appallingly high, and women were afraid of dying in childbirth. Infant mortality was high, too. One in ten babies were born sick or dead.

Today 99 percent of deliveries are in a hospital, and the birth attendant is usually an obstetrician. Medical management, which means leaving all decisions in the doctor's hands, also is routine in most hospital deliveries, although many doctors do discuss procedures carefully with patients before going ahead. Our maternal mortality rate has plummeted eight- or tenfold and is among the lowest in the world, despite the estimation that 10 to 15 percent of American mothers have inadequate prenatal care. Infant mortality has been halved, and even though our infant mortality rate is only the fifteenth lowest in the world, only one in twenty babies, or 5 percent, is born sick or dead. We still have a long way to go to reduce infant mortality, but obstetricians and anesthesiologists are very proud of the achievements of the past quarter-century and feel they have come about because of the development and implementation of high safety standards by both doctors and hospitals.

What price safety? Despite the improved statistics, many people contend that hospitals are too impersonal and rigid, depriving the mother of her individuality and fulfillment. They advocate restoring the emotional supports and personal freedom that make childbirth a satisfying experience.

Little by little, the old regulations *are* being reevaluated and changed by hospitals, partly in response to consumer demands expressed individually and through such national organizations as the International Childbirth Education Association (ICEA), which began twenty-five years ago in the Midwest. Doctors are beginning to recognize both as individuals and through their professional organizations that hospital childbirth must become more family centered and emotionally satisfying.

Before they go to a hospital, most women have no idea what routines they will encounter or how they will react to them. Therefore, they are in no position to decide which they can live with and which may prove intolerable. If you learn about these routines and gauge your own reactions to them beforehand, you will be in a position to make special requests of your doctor and hospital, or to make a better selection of a hospital setting. That more sympathetic setting may prove to be a distance away, but, as Doris Olson, president of the ICEA, points out, "For years, people have been traveling distances to get the childbirth experience they want."

You should also know about the new innovations before you go to the hospital to deliver. Electronic fetal monitoring, a technique that has become common only in the last few years, is routinely used in about 25 percent of hospitals, mainly the larger medical centers that can afford this expensive equipment for all deliveries. There are also many new testing procedures for diagnosing fetal abnormalities and, in the near future, doctors will be feeding, diagnosing, and operating on babies even before they are born!

Some researchers look forward to the day when we will be able to diagnose all fetuses with these procedures before birth, treating those that are salvageable and aborting those that are not, to prevent most birth defects. They feel that the combination of electronic fetal monitoring and routine testing will greatly reduce stillbirths, mental retardation, and the neurological damage that may be caused by the birth process. Their reason for routine monitoring is that one-third of all problems occur during labor to apparently healthy, low-risk mothers.

I believe that every mother-to-be should be aware of the reasons for and the advantages of the new procedures, as well as their side effects and risks, which are causing controversy. It is often difficult to insist on being an exception to hospital routines and regulations, but parents do have a definite choice in the case of the new procedures because usually they must give permission in writing before a test can be performed. This chapter will help you raise the questions that need to be satisfactorily answered before you give consent. For the more hazardous procedures, I suggest that you seek a second, independent, qualified opinion so you can feel satisfied that you are doing everything you can to advance and protect your own and your baby's health.

THE HOSPITAL EXPERIENCE

Except in a handful of situations, routine medical interventions are performed by medical personnel on *every* mother admitted to a hospital for childbirth.

It is vitally important that you thoroughly understand their use. The criteria for using the newer routines is still highly controversial in American obstetrics. Here, for example, is the assessment of Dr. Frederick Ettner, of the American College of Home Obstetrics in Chicago, who feels that their indications have become dangerously broad and routine:

"Obstetrical care in the United States has evolved, in the last decade, into a technology of scientific medical obstetrics. . . . Normal physiological functions have become abnormal. The extreme and exceptional obstetrical cases have become the mean and the rule, respectively. Full normal development is rapidly approaching obscurity."

But is the point of view of Dr. Stanley James, professor of Pediatrics, Obstetrics, and Gynecology at Columbia University College of Physicians and Surgeons, more correct? "Each of these developments offers special benefits for mother and infant when used correctly. There is an important place for each of these interventions if there are specific maternal or fetal indications."

Let us look at each of the routines closely.

The Hospital Routines

Most women have their pubic hair shaved and are given an enema to empty their bowels upon entering the labor room. The rationale for these procedures is that they provide protection against infection after episiotomy (cutting of the area between the vagina and the anus) and permit the baby to pass through the maternal pelvis more easily.

Natural-childbirth advocates are questioning these time-honored procedures, which add to the disconcerting sickroom atmosphere of a hospital delivery and are almost universally hated by women. A woman entering a hospital often is feeling frightened and uncomfortable with beginning contractions. Separated from her husband, she is whisked into a new and stressful experience. In the hands of strange nurses and house staff, she feels emotionally vulnerable to any procedure that adds to her feelings of powerlessness, of being manipulated.

Some studies report that shaving the pubic area actually creates a higher incidence of infection in that region, and it is an experience that is highly unpleasant for most women. The stubble of hair growth afterward is irritating and disturbing to the woman's feelings about her sexual attractiveness, already weakened after childbirth.

Enemas, which are given in order to empty the pelvis and make room for the baby, have sometimes caused contractions to become stronger and harder to control. These, in turn, can incline a woman to ask for drug relief.

Doctors usually advise women not to eat once labor begins, since it can result in complications if anesthesia is administered. Yet prolonged fasting has been found to be bad for both mother and baby. Therefore, IVs are attached for intravenous feeding. Unfortunately, recent research indicates this solution may be dangerous for a sick baby, besides being uncomfortable, even painful, for the mother. Psychologically, an IV is associated with being sick, and the mother attached to one will tend to stay immobile in order not to jar the needle. Midwives and doctors in home deliveries encourage the mother to eat lightly if labor is prolonged. They have not found that vomiting during labor, which occurs occasionally, is harmful to a healthy mother who is not medicated.

COMMON DELIVERY PROCEDURES

Forceps or Vacuum Extractor

Forceps or a vacuum extractor (the latter is used less often because of its disadvantages) are employed to remove a baby "expeditiously" when distress is noted. Studies indicate that these procedures are used in about 65 percent of American hospital deliveries today.

Advocates maintain the forceps are a great advantage under special circumstances. For example, it is considered good medical practice to deliver premature babies by elective low forceps to spare them from having their heads compressed against the mother's perineum. Also, in Dr. James's opinion, "Forceps can be less dangerous than a cesarean section, which has the potential hazard of anesthetic complications and more postnatal infections."

Natural-childbirth advocates point out that forceps are so commonly required because the routine medicating of the mother interferes with her voluntary efforts to expel her baby.

The higher the forceps, the more dangerous the delivery. Even mid forceps have been replaced by cesarean section. Still, there are dangers even in mid-low forceps. These include increased incidence of hemorrhage to the baby's head, damage to facial nerves, and the possibility of other neurological impairment. Doris Haire also cautions, "No one knows the degree of compression or traction a fetal head can tolerate before sustaining brain damage."

Episiotomy

Episiotomy, an incision made into the perineum between the vaginal opening and anus to facilitate delivery of the baby, is routine in American hospital childbirth. This procedure is much less frequently done in home births here, or in hospital and home births abroad.

Most obstetricians believe that this simple incision prevents tearing, which is difficult to repair when it is extensive, and that it thus helps restore women's bodies to their normal size and sexual function sooner.

Natural-childbirth advocates counter that it is the usual position of American hospital childbirth—flat on the back, knees up and spread wide apart—that creates the need for episiotomies to prevent tearing. They have found that episiotomies are largely unnecessary when the mother is allowed to move around freely, particularly when she delivers in a vertical or squatting position, taking advantage of the force of gravity. Pelvic floor exercises during pregnancy and oil massage of the area during labor also have been found to reduce the incidence of tearing. When tearing does occur in home births, it is usually small enough to heal easily without stitches, or with only one or two stitches.

In the view of many childbirth and sex experts, the muscle tissue severed in episiotomy is permanently weakened and the stitch-up can cause problems, particularly if it is done too tightly. The incision itself is hardly painful, since the area is numb from pressure. However, pain is common during the healing period, and this weakens a woman's sexual self-confidence and desire so that she tends to put off resuming sex longer than she would if she had not had an episiotomy.

Sheila Kitzinger has found that some women experience episiotomy as a sexual assault and suffer from spasms during intercourse afterward. As a sex therapist, I frequently hear about sexual problems after episiotomy. Some women report pain during intercourse that lasts for many months, even years. Others feel that their normal ability to have orgasm has been impaired. Some women accommodate by having sex in a rear-entry position, but if this change inhibits them or is less fulfilling than the frontal, embracing position, they feel permanently handi-capped.

Although these are subjective reports, they are heard so frequently that it seems wise to avoid having a routine episiotomy, and to work at repair afterward if you do have one. Here are some guidelines regarding episiotomies:

1. Find a doctor who is willing to deliver you without a routine episiotomy and who will not cut until he is sure it is necessary.

2. Ask the doctor not to put your legs in stirrups since a more natural position helps prevent tearing. Any position that takes advantage of the force of gravity is greatly preferable to a supine position.

3. Some doctors and midwives use oil or vitamin E massage of the perineum during delivery because they believe it helps prevent tearing.

1. Do your pelvic floor exercises during pregnancy, and resume them directly after immediate postpartum recovery. (See Chapter II for directions.) You will feel some discomfort from the stitches, but the exercises will help alleviate it. Your circulation will increase, which helps to heal not only the episiotomy but also the hemorrhoids or other varicose veins caused by pregnancy, labor, and the pressure of delivery.

5. Use tub baths, icepacks, infrared lamps, analgesic sprays, or lubrication ointment to help healing.

Stirrups and the Supine Position

By now you are probably questioning the position to use in labor and delivery. Good!

It may surprise you to learn that, throughout history, lying flat on one's back, with feet in stirrups and knees up and spread apart, has hard-ly been the favored position for a woman having a baby. Women have walked about during labor, lain on their sides in a favorite sleep position, or sat up, supported by their husbands, friends, or a solid backrest. Many still use a squatting position for delivery. Dr. Caldeyro Barcia, president of the International Federation of Obstetricians and Gynecologists, has said that "except for being hanged by the feet, the supine [flat-on-the-back] position is the worst conceivable position for labor and delivery." It is the least comfortable, slows down uterine activity, and adversely affects the maintenance of normal blood pressure in labor. He adds:

"When the mother is in the supine position, it's harder for the head to come into the birth canal. In an extensive study comparing low-risk women in twenty-one countries, those who stood or walked about had a considerably shorter labor and were more comfortable sitting or standing than lying down. Contractions are stronger in the vertical position, and blocking of blood to the baby by pressure on the umbilical cord can be corrected simply by changing the mother's position. And, of course, episiotomies are more frequently needed when the mother is in a supine position."

A woman need not lie passively on her back during labor and delivery. Giving birth can be a joyful activity for both parents! (Dr. David Kliot/Brookdale Hospital Medical Center)

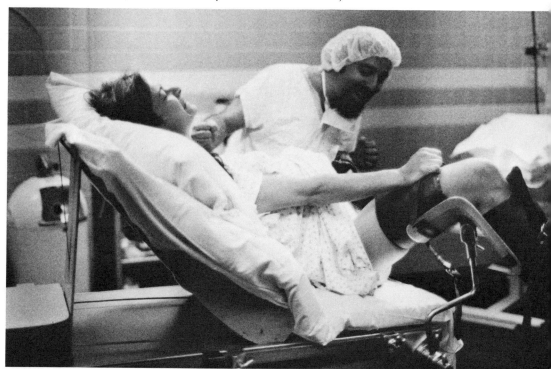

In her booklet *The Cultural Warping of Childbirth*, Doris Haire talks about the complicated consequences that may ensue from assuming the supine position in labor and delivery:

> It adversely affects the mother's blood pressure, cardiac return and pulmonary ventilation; decreases the normal intensity of contraction; inhibits the mother's involuntary efforts to push her baby out spontaneously; increases the need for forceps and increases the traction necessary for forceps extraction. . . . [It] increases the need for episiotomy because of increased tension on the pelvic floor. . . . Normal separation of the feet for natural expulsion of the baby is 15–16 inches, which is far less than is allowed by the average American delivery table stirrups.

Because of the known advantages of other birth positions, some hospitals are changing their practices and allowing mothers to lean on backrests or lie in beds that have sections that can be raised or lowered. But these changes are coming slowly and hard. Dr. Daniel Friedman of Long Island reports his experience in trying to introduce his own backrest chair into the delivery room: "The nurses kept washing the chair, worrying about whether it was sterile enough. There was so much objection, misplacing of the chair, etc., that I had to give up."

Explore with your doctor how you can avoid the flat-on-the-back position in the labor and delivery rooms, and ask him not to use the stirrups and not to strap your arms in delivery. If you insist, he may arrange an exception of some or all of these routines.

MEDICAL INTERVENTIONS

Within the last decade, new procedures have been developed that have revolutionized hospital childbirth. Like all medical procedures, they offer advantages but carry risks. Therefore, they should be applied *only* when medically indicated and not for the convenience of the physician or the mother. Let's take a look at them:

Oxytocin to Induce Labor

The hormone oxytocin, which is secreted by the posterior pituitary gland, stimulates labor. The quality and quantity of contractions are greatly affected when synthetic oxytocin is infused—very often contractions are stronger and longer, with shorter relaxation periods between.

This may be bad for the baby, according to Dr. Ettner: "The fetus may be stressed before its first breath. The frequency and strength of contractions decrease the ability of the fetus to restore its supply of oxygen. With each strong contraction, the blood supply to the uterus is temporarily shut off." Indeed, a study by Dr. Barry Shifrin of Cedars of Lebanon Hospital, in Los Angeles, found that when oxytocin was given to women in labor, 25 percent showed some asphyxiation patterns, and when oxytocin and epidural anesthesia were used together, 50 percent showed such patterns.

According to Dr. Caldeyro-Barcia, "in less than 2 percent of deliveries is oxytocin needed to induce labor, and yet in 40 to 50 percent of deliveries it is used."

When oxytocin is used to speed labor, because of the increased strength of contractions, a pain-killing drug or anesthesia is much more likely to be needed. Also, oxytocin's rate of success is only 85 percent, which means that sometimes labor will stop in the middle, with the mother partly dilated. Being sent home in this condition and told to return to the hospital when labor begins normally is a harrowing experience, I can tell you personally.

Induction of Labor by Rupturing the Membranes

Early rupturing of the sac (the membranes) in which the baby lies is performed to shorten labor or to induce it. Though it has been a very common procedure for years, it is not without hazards and side effects.

Instead of the normal, wavelike contractions of natural labor, induced labor contractions reach full intensity rapidly and remain intense. There is no question that labor is shorter, and your doctor may feel this is important to avoid fetal distress. The major risks to be considered are uterine rupture and a prolapse (falling out of its normal position) of the umbilical cord. Even if these conditions do not occur, according to Dr. Caldeyro-Barcia, there is this consideration: "Early rupture can damage the baby's brain and cause marked disturbance in the skin and brain circulation. . . . The first stage of labor is shortened, but at the cost of the deformation of the baby's head. Spontaneous rupture usually occurs in advanced labor. The time of rupture strongly influences the duration of labor, but leaves the fetal head unprotected. There also is a marked fall in the fetal heartbeat when the membranes are ruptured."

Doctors differ in their thinking about when induction is indicated.

Ask your doctor for his position on this question. Certainly, he should never induce the baby to suit his weekend or vacation convenience, which, believe it or not, is frequently done. There is a risk of overestimating the fetus's maturity, and that may result in a premature baby.

Induction of the "Overdue" Baby

Though only 5 percent of first babies come on the "due date," mothers and doctors begin to grow restless after it passes, thinking the baby may be "postmature"—or what mothers call "late." The risk of postmaturity is that the placenta might be deteriorating, becoming more and more inadequate to support the baby. The doctor frequently will suggest an "oxytocin challenge test" (described below) to see if the baby would be able to tolerate natural labor, or he may try to induce the baby by one of the measures already described.

As with all interventions, there are abuses. Here's what Dr. Robert Bradley, developer of the Bradley method of childbirth preparation, has to say about overconcern with the "due date": "If you take all the eight-pound babies that had spontaneous labor without induction, you'll find that 80 percent of them were born after that stupid 'due date.' That's because doctors count from the last menstrual period rather than from conception."

When you're "overdue," and both you and your doctor are worrying about hurrying up your delivery, is hardly the time to debate the pros and cons of induction. I suggest you discuss the whole question in a series of interviews with obstetricians before selecting the one to work with. "Excessive" weight gain (discussed in chapter 2) and induction because the baby is "late" are the two issues that most frequently disturb otherwise normal and happy pregnancies and childbirths. Why not choose a doctor whose philosophy about these issues matches your own?

Oxytocin Challenge Test

Oxytocin also is used to predict how well a baby will do in labor. Dr. Ettner explains the procedure and its use: "The oxytocin challenge test, also called 'stressed monitoring,' consists of observing the fetal heart rate in response to induced uterine contractions. It is currently widely used as a prenatal screening for successful labor and delivery of high-risk patients. However, the definition of 'high-risk' is continually being broadened. The test attempts to duplicate the stresses of labor by inducing contractions and observing the fetal heart response so that placental reserve and fetal welfare can be evaluated."

Criteria for the test now include prolonged pregnancy (more than forty-two weeks based on the estimated date of conception), staining, previous stillbirths, and concern that the baby may not be strong enough to withstand normal labor.

"Typically, OCT is performed late in pregnancy, from the thirty-first through the forty-fourth week. Synthetic oxytocin is infused through the vein, with increasing doses every ten to twenty minutes until frequent uterine contractions are elicited. This is continued for twenty minutes with electronic fetal monitoring. If the baby's heart doesn't recover properly between the contractions, this is considered a sign that the baby is under stress." However, Dr. Ettner does not feel that this is necessarily so. He says, "Studies have shown that 25 percent of patients with positive OCTs when allowed to labor normally, deliver without complication. OCT has been a disappointing way of predicting the subsequent performance of the fetus in labor, yet OCTs have been promoted to the point of a self-fulfilling prophecy."

Medical opinion about the value and risk of using OCT remains divided. Some doctors are concerned that the hormone oxytocin might itself have an adverse effect on the fetus. A Mexican cardiologist and pediatrician has recently developed an alternate stress test that uses maternal exercise in combination with ultrasonic monitoring of the fetus to determine its state of well-being.

Many others are convinced of OCT's values, including some natural-childbirth advocates like Theresa Dundero, nurse-midwife at Albert Einstein Hospital in New York. She says, "Statistics at my hospital show that 80 percent of babies who have a positive stress go on to problems in labor." Therefore, she recommends the test to those of her patients who are sure their conception dates were more than forty-two weeks earlier.

Before agreeing to OCT, it is wise to get a second opinion. After the test is performed is hardly the time to resist the medical recommendations that follow.

Amniocentesis

Amniocentesis is the sampling of the amniotic fluid to detect abnormalities in the fetus or to judge its maturity. By means of a long hollow needle inserted through the abdomen, a sample of amniotic fluid can be removed for analysis. Then the sex of the baby can be determined, and whether the fetus is likely to inherit a sex-linked disorder such as hemophilia or muscular dystrophy. The age of the fetus and the maturity of its lungs can be ascertained. A chromosome count can be made, which diagnoses certain types of defects, including mental retardation and severe physical handicaps. Chemical composition studies reveal possible enzyme deficiencies, which can create serious digestive or respiratory diseases and whether an Rh baby needs intrauterine transfusion to survive.

Some childbirth experts and obstetricians recommend amniocentesis for all pregnancies where the mother is over thirty-five. It has been found that, with a mother under thirty-five, the risk of mongolism, or Down's syndrome, is only one in two thousand births. Between thirty-five and forty, the risk is one in five hundred births, and over forty, it is one in one hundred births. Obviously, amniocentesis is one of the major advances in obstetrics.

Still, amniocentesis itself offers serious risk. Usually, the test is done at sixteen weeks, to detect possible abnormalities with an eye to aborting the baby if they are found. Close to the end of pregnancy, the procedure is performed when induced delivery is contemplated, to predict the likelihood of respiratory distress due to lung immaturity.

The enormous benefit of sparing parents the burden of raising seriously handicapped youngsters should never be underestimated. But it is equally important that a mother recognize the risks of amniocentesis, which include placental hemorrhage, blood exchange of mother and baby (creating greater Rh incompatibility while testing for it), serious bleeding or injury to a vital part of the baby. There can be infection of the amniotic fluid, leakage of the fluid, peritonitis, blood clots, and vague abdominal pains.

Dr. Ettner observes, "The procedure can save a life, but when it becomes routine, it is being misused. Despite tragic outcomes, some doctors are counseling liberal use." He points out that consent forms for amniocentesis, which parents must sign before it can be performed, state that the doctor and hospital are released from responsibility if the procedure causes any damage to the mother or fetus, or if it initiates premature labor, which can result in spontaneous abortion. The forms also say that the attempt to get the fluid may be unsuccessful, and a correct diagnosis cannot be guaranteed.

Doris Haire discusses what this release form means for the patient: "Most release forms are just attempts to relieve the doctor of liability. However, unless the mother is given a full explanation of the risks and hazards and pertinent areas of uncertainty, neither the physician nor the hospital is released from legal liability."

I trust that you are already convinced never to have amniocentesis merely to determine the sex of your baby! And I hope that you will never agree to the procedure without fully exploring the reasons. Discuss with your doctor the whole procedure and why he feels it's needed in your situation. Get a second opinion. Your decision about whether to proceed will then be based on a serious consideration of whether the benefit outweighs the risk. The decision and the consequences both belong to you.

Ultrasound

Originally developed for the space program, ultrasound is a procedure that either projects a sound picture, recording the placement of the placenta and fetus inside the uterus, or monitors the fetal heart rate. Since X-rays now are considered dangerous, ultrasound is being used instead. There are hand devices and fixed ones, attached to an electronic fetal monitor (see page 67), with which ultrasound is used. Sometimes ultrasound is used early in pregnancy, to check the fetal heart rate during routine examinations or to locate the fetus when amniocentesis is being considered. Most often it is used during labor, as part of monitoring.

Ultrasound is used to detect developmental disorders, identify multiple pregnancies, chart fetal growth, and make diagnoses of many possible abnormalities of pregnancy or in the mother.

The major problem with ultrasound is that it is still so new that we won't know its long-range effects for years. In 1977, the U. S. Food and Drug Administration initiated a long-term follow-up study to determine whether or not ultrasound has adverse effects on human development. Animal studies indicate that diagnostic levels of ultrasound—one and a half to five minutes' exposure—can disrupt the spleen's ability to produce antibodies, disturbing the immunological system. There may be other adverse consequences.

Doris Haire, who is a member of the U.. S. Food and Drug Administration's Committee on Fetal Monitoring, says, "There is growing concern among scientists that ultrasound may prove harmful to the vulnerable ova of the female fetus. A woman is born with all the ova she'll ever have. Whether these will produce healthy children may be affected by ultrasonic radiation used on her while she was still a fetus." However, Dr. Finster points out that another study of several generations of mice that were subjected to prolonged diagnostic levels of ultrasound failed to show any damage to the reproductive cells of either sex. Unfortunately, no animal study can duplicate human response exactly.

"Meanwhile," Ms. Haire advises, "it would seem common sense to use ultrasound devices only when medically indicated. Those who contend that ultrasound used for fetal monitoring is harmless should be reminded that many men and women now have cancer as a result of X-ray therapy for acne, enlarged tonsils, etc., because X-rays were once considered harmless.

Electronic Fetal Monitoring (EFM)

Read this section carefully, since your decision about EFM will determine your choice of hospital and possibly also your choice of doctor or midwife to help you deliver your baby.

EFM is revolutionizing American childbirth. It was developed by two groups of physicians, one headed by Dr. Caldeyro-Barcia in Montevideo, Uruguay and the other, in this country, by Dr. Edward H. G. Hon beginning in 1955 at Yale University. Although EFM has only been available for common use in the past five or six years, 25 percent of hospital births today are electronically monitored. Many doctors are so enthusiastic about EFM that they look forward to the time when 100 percent of American childbirths will be electronically monitored (that rate already exists in some of our large medical centers). The states of New York and California at one time even considered mandating electronic monitoring for all deliveries.

Advocates of EFM are sure that its use is reducing the incidence of stillbirths, mental retardation, and neurological damage. They believe these tragedies happen frequently and unexpectedly, and that constant electronic monitoring of the fetus's heartbeat is a clearly effective means of prevention. Dr. James points out, "In 10 percent of all deliveries, complications develop that cannot be anticipated beforehand."

The reason advocates prefer EFM to listening to the heartbeat through a stethoscope (called auscultation) is that the human ear is fallible, and the recording of the tracing is as important for diagnosis as the beat itself. Others are just as passionate in their denunciation of electronic monitoring. When no drugs or anesthesia is used, they point out, unexpected tragedies don't occur so frequently or so quickly that auscultation won't pick them up efficiently.

A study by the Department of Reproductive Biology at Case-Western Reserve University School of Medicine found that 41 percent of patients could not even be monitored successfully. The reasons? Patients were uncooperative, catheters became dislodged, fetal-scalp electrodes got displaced, and electronic equipment failed. Their conclusion was that "electronic fetal monitoring should be reserved for the high-risk patient."

Dr. Ettner described the problems that can arise in using EFM: "Sometimes the *maternal* heart rate is recorded by mistake. Since it's only half as fast as the baby's, this can lead to panic in the labor room, with mothers getting upset by the flashing lights and sound of the equipment. One-fourth of the women complain of pain and discomfort, particularly when the equipment is inserted. The incidence of infection of the uterus afterward is higher when the monitor is used. Insertion requires rupture of the waters, and amniotic fluids can become infected.

Recent studies by Albert D. Havercamp, director of Perinatal Research at Denver General Hospital in Denver, Colorado, show that there are no differences in outcome for infants monitored by nurse or machine, except one—machine monitoring results in an almost tripling of cesarean section rate. He says, "Five or six years ago doctors questioned EFM, but now they would be forlorn without monitors. Obstetricians are very vulnerable to criticism. They have a sincere desire to improve infant outcome and feel in scientific control. But EFM is *not* a must. It has a very small place in obstetrics."

Yet a large study in England in 1973 showed that infant mortality fell with electronic fetal monitoring. Dr. Hon, who is now continuing his work at the University of Southern California in Los Angeles, with Dr.

Richard Paul found in 1970 that proper use of EFM *reduced* cesarean section by 7 percent in their hospital. Advocates now are pointing to a recent Australian study, by Dr. Peter Renou and associates of the Queen Victoria Memorial Hospital, Melbourne, Australia. Despite a small rise in C-section rate in their high-risk monitored patients, the number of babies needing intensive care afterward was higher in the auscultated group. Although they caution that their work cannot be used to draw general conclusions because of differences in medical standards throughout the world, they do feel EFM is necessary and warranted for high-risk patients at their hospital. In regard to criticisms about patients' negative emotional reactions to EFM, they claim, "Many women suffer anxiety concerning the welfare of the fetus *in utero* and it would seem likely that monitoring, properly explained to the patient, would reduce maternal anxiety."

This conclusion is highly questionable. Most mothers in normal, low-risk situations, do not worry about the possible ill health of their baby during labor and delivery, unless they have deep-seated anxieties about producing a defective child. It is more reasonable to conclude that in *normal* pregnancies, EFM might arouse unnecessary anxiety, whereas in high-risk situations, where the mother already knows the infant is in jeopardy, the same procedure would be reassuring.

Are these interventions (IV, EFM) routinely necessary? (R. P. Sheridan/Columbia-Presbyterian Medical Center)

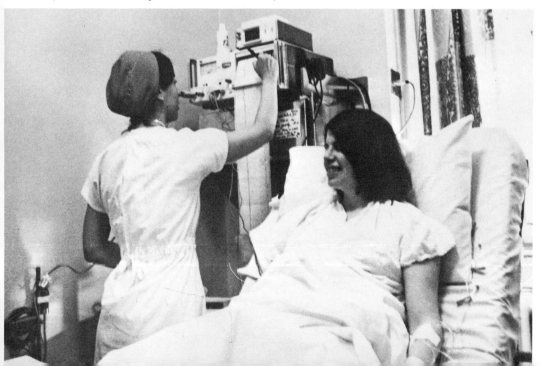

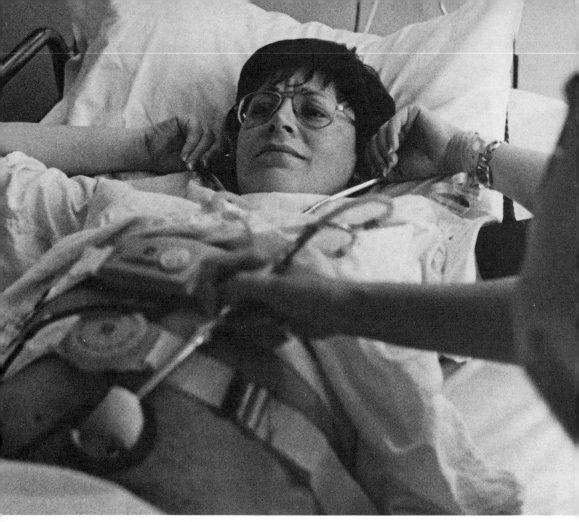

The external fetal monitor is used early in labor, before the waters break, to check the baby's heartbeat. (Alison Ehrlich Wachstein, from Pregnant Moments, Morgan & Morgan, 1978)

The paraphernalia of the hospital labor room can seem overwhelming, especially if you don't learn about it in advance. (R.P. Sheridan/Columbia-Presbyterian Medical Center)

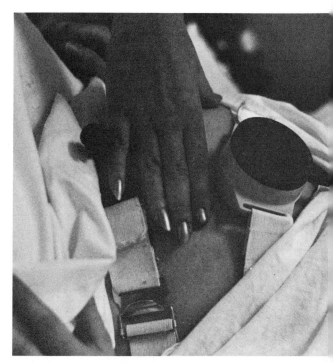

Doctors who question the routine use of EFM believe that its major advantage is the time saved by hospital personnel, since it permits monitoring of babies from a centrally located station where nurses can see at a glance what is happening by looking at the machine. They feel that doctors and nurses are losing their ability to make a diagnosis without resorting to data from the machine. Dr. Jacqueline Hott of the Adelphi School of Nursing, Long Island, New York, told me, "EFM removes the human touch. A patient told me the doctor didn't look at her once. He just fiddled with the machinery."

Advocates counter that the use of monitors is realistic, permitting better supervision of laboring women by the nursing personnel available.

Dr. Ettner describes the procedure for inserting internal monitors: "Electronic monitoring is facilitated only in active labor, after a cervical dilation of 2 to 3 centimeters, and after rupture of the fetal membranes. Two sterile catheters containing electronic leads to the monitor are manually placed. One lead punctures the fetal scalp via a spiral electrode and relays the fetal cardiogram. The other lies between the fetus and the wall of the uterus and relays the rate and relative pressure of uterine contractions."

Because the internal monitors require rupturing of the membranes, most often an external monitor is used in early labor. There are two types of external monitors, one using ultrasound and the other using electrodes glued to the maternal abdomen. In addition, another sensor is strapped to the abdomen, recording the intensity and frequency of uterine contractions. As labor proceeds, women feel increasingly uncomfortable with external monitoring because of the pressure of the straps and the way they limit movement. When the monitor is on a cart, the woman can sit in a chair as well as lie in bed, but in most situations, it is a standing machine that is attached to a woman lying down.

What about possible complications for the baby? "Ten percent of babies get scalp hematomas [black and blue marks]. They also get scalp abcesses and cellulitis. There can be spinal fluid leakage," reports Dr. Ettner.

An important reason to question the value of EFM in normal, low-risk situations is the unprecedented rise in cesarean births that has accompanied it. There is evidence that medical personnel may be overreacting to normal fluctuations in fetal heartbeat and considering them signs of fetal distress. Dr. Finster, an advocate of fetal monitoring in labor, points out that, "Monitoring is indeed a science, and people should know how to use it and make proper interpretations." Still, according to Dr. Havercamp, "We are too arbitrary in terminating pregnancies that are electronically monitored."

Also, because the membranes must be ruptured before the internal monitor can be attached, the device may be creating the very conditions of distress it is designed to monitor. Says Dr. Ettner, "During labor, following the spontaneous rupture of the membranes, every uterine contraction causes a transient decrease in the fetal heart. . . . This is of no consequence, except when the rupture of the membranes is artificially effected early in the first stage of labor. With the early artificial rupture, the fetal head is defenseless. Decreases in the fetal heart rate can then result in fetal distress. Not only can EFM alert physicians to fetal distress, monitoring can *cause* fetal distress. Truly, the fetus has been challenged. The EFM dutifully records the stressed fetal heart rate. With suspicions confirmed, a diagnosis of fetal distress is noted and elective cesarean section is the treatment of choice."

Dr. David Stewart, co-founder of NAPSAC (National Association of Parents and Professionals for Safe Alternatives in Childbirth), an organization that alerts the public to possible dangers of the new interventions (see Part Three), feels strongly that "Women should refuse to be part of an experiment." Doris Haire advises that before you consent to the procedure, you ask the doctor to sign a form agreeing to be responsible for any harm or injury that may result to the baby from EFM or ultrasound.

Because of all this controversy, some women prefer to be monitored by a nurse or doctor rather than the machine. Yet they want to be in a setting where EFM is available should anything go wrong. That requires finding a doctor who will go along with your preferences, and a setting that will permit him to apply EFM only when there is a deviation from normality. Some hospitals, particularly those with midwife units, do operate this way. ICEA or ASPO (see Appendices I and II) will refer you to a hospital where electronic fetal monitoring is reserved for problem situations.

5

The Cesarean
Birth Experience

WHAT IS A CESAREAN BIRTH?

According to legend, Julius Caesar was delivered abdominally, and so the procedure bears his name. The problem with this legend is that in those days it was nearly always fatal to have surgery. Yet Caesar's mother is supposed to have lived for many years after his birth! However the procedure *is* very old; it is mentioned both in the Talmud and in seventeenth-century medical literature.

Once it became possible to control infection with antiseptics (around 1865), abdominal surgery did become an alternative to difficult vaginal delivery. Now that we have germ-free surgery, cesarean delivery has become one of the safest of all major operations. In the last decade, its use has increased fivefold in America. Whenever possible, the operation is performed on the lower, thinned-out muscle tissue of the uterus rather than the thick, contracting middle section, which decreases the possibility that the uterus will rupture in subsequent pregnancies. While it is no longer necessary for a woman who has had a cesarean section to deliver all subsequent children by this method, previous C-section is the most frequent reason that cesareans are being done today.

There are indications that the rate of cesareans will continue to rise as the operation changes from one of necessity to one of choice. The basic reason is a shift of priorities from the mother to the fetus; that is, the emphasis is now on sparing the fetus any trouble whatever in being born. Medical experts say, "You get pregnant to have a healthy baby, not a vaginal delivery. We are looking for a neurologically and psychologically sound human being now. In an advanced country, we expect a baby to survive."

While there are no absolute criteria for performing cesareans, here are the sorts of emergencies that indicate its use: when the placenta is partially or completely detached from the uterine wall (abruption); when the umbilical cord hangs from the vagina (prolapse); when the placenta is blocking the birth canal (placenta previa); when infection follows from too-early rupturing of the membranes before labor begins. In these situations, C-section has saved many lives.

Some illnesses of the mother also call for its use: if the mother has hypertension or diabetes, particularly if the fetus is large; if she has an infected vagina; if she has toxemia of pregnancy. Mother-fetus incompatibilities in Rh factor or disproportion between the mother's pelvis and the baby's head are also clear indications for C-section to be performed.

The "elective" reasons are rising. The most common one is repeat cesarean—the mother had one previously. Other reasons concern the baby: the doctor may feel vaginal delivery will be too difficult for the baby if stress tests indicate the heartbeat is weak, or if the baby's position is breech, particularly in a first delivery. Today a primapara (first-time mother) has about a one-in-four chance of delivering her baby abdominally.

DISADVANTAGES OF A CESAREAN BIRTH

Even though the outcome of cesareans is generally good, most doctors agree that the operation carries risks and disadvantages. Dr. Gerald G. Anderson, chief of Obstetrics at Yale–New Haven Medical School, has outlined these: "A cesarean is a major operation. It necessitates the risk of a general anesthetic. There is a risk in any major abdominal surgery from bleeding, clots, etc. . . . The mother is left with a scar on her uterus; that weakens it. The next time she gets pregnant, the uterus could rupture before labor, during labor, or during delivery, and rupture carries a very high mortality rate for the mother and the baby. We have to think about how many children the woman wants after this birth. If she's going to have more children, a cesarean will complicate her life, and she will be a sort of obstetric cripple from that day on."

Cesarean nurse Ruth Allen notes that half the mothers are nauseated enough after the operation to require oxygen. There is postoperative pain, and many women suffer from gas pains.

Dr. Michael Bergman, of the New York Infirmary in Manhattan, points to the heavy responsibility on the doctor. First of all, elective cesareans must be delicately timed: definite criteria must be met to make sure the baby is developed enough to be delivered without risk of prematurity, and the operation should never be done earlier than ten to fourteen days before the expected confinement. Secondly, once intervention is begun, good timing again is of the utmost importance to avoid the ill effects of surgical handling on the mother and baby and to spare the baby the effects of anesthesia to the greatest extent possible.

Cesareans cost about $1000 more than a normal delivery. You will have to stay in the hospital for a week or ten days and then make arrangements for help with the baby when you return home. Also, breast-feeding is much more difficult. You may need postoperative painkillers, which will keep you asleep a lot of the time.

Your scar will take up to six weeks to heal, and during the first few weeks, you will experience a great deal of fatigue. During your recuperation, it is important to avoid such physical stresses as long drives, stair climbing, and heavy household chores. This is usual after any surgery, but many mothers do not expect these aftereffects or plan for sufficient help at home so they can recuperate comfortably.

CONTROVERSY ABOUT ELECTIVE CESAREANS

Because of the rapidly rising rate of cesareans, there is growing concern that the operation is being elected too liberally. Repeat cesarean is under increasing attack, and many doctors believe each case should be reviewed on its own merits. In other countries—England, for example— that a woman has had a previous cesarean is not reason enough for performing one again.

The liveliest medical disagreement is about whether breech position is a sufficient reason to perform a cesarean, even with a first baby. Admittedly, breech deliveries are more difficult and can be considered "high-risk," yet many mothers and babies come through normal delivery with excellent results.

Dr. Frederick Ettner discusses research findings on breech and C-section: "In an analysis of five hundred cases of breech, most patients delivered vaginally with little or no difficulty. Cesarean section was found justifiable 12 to 15 percent of the time. Another study described a method of studying the patient with breech presentation prior to delivery. An evaluation of certain factors in the patient's history and physical examination enabled them to predict, with a high degree of accuracy, the outcome of a breech delivery. Cesarean section was indicated in only 15 percent of the high-risk breech group and 4 percent of the low-risk breech group."

A second concern is whether "fetal distress" is being diagnosed too quickly now because of the widespread use of the electronic fetal monitor. Dr. Albert Havercamp has conducted large-scale research with high-risk mothers in which half were monitored by machine and half by nurses using stethescopes. He found that the only difference in outcome was that almost three times as many C-sections were ordered for the machine-monitored mothers. Dr. Finster suggests, "There are trigger-happy people who will intervene as soon as the baby's heartbeat goes down on the electronic monitor." He questions whether EFM is *causing* the rise in C-sections.

Your choice of a doctor can be a determining factor in whether cesarean section is likely to be employed in elective situations like breech or twin delivery. If the baby is premature or overdue, one doctor may elect to do a cesarean to spare the baby the stress of a vaginal delivery while another may not. If your doctor is likely to use an oxytocin challenge test rather than wait out a "late" baby, the chances of cesarean are greater. If an elective decision is made for cesarean, natural-childbirth advocates suggest you get a second opinion before agreeing to the procedure.

POSSIBLE LONG-TERM EFFECTS

We have talked about some of the advantages and disadvantages of cesareans, when they are life-saving and necessary, and how they spare the baby the ordeal of a difficult vaginal delivery. Recent research by a few psychologists and psychiatrists shows that there may be longer term effects on the baby's development. I must emphasize that these findings are very new and are considered highly speculative at this point. Nonetheless, if they hold up, they should lead to further evaluations on the frequent use of cesarean in elective situations.

Cultural anthropologist and author Ashley Montagu recently reviewed these findings in a lecture in Los Angeles before the Primal Foundation. Here is what he says:

Babies born abdominally may be missing vital tactile stimulation of a normal womb delivery. The substitute for [an animal's] licking is labor, during which there are massive contractions on the body of the fetus. There are Cesarean children born who have had no labor whatever. If these children have not been adequately stimulated by the contractions of the uterus you would expect that they would suffer from inadequacies of the gastrointestinal, genital-urinary and respiratory tracts. And this is exactly what you find. When these children were put to bowel and bladder training they had gastro-intestinal inadequacies. They also are notoriously subject to upper respiratory tract infection during the first two years of their lives and tend to be shallow breathers.

Psychologist-author Arthur Janov, in *The Feeling Child,* goes further:

Cesarean babies are more emotionally disturbed . . . more fearful and restless. In response to stimuli they tend to be more passive. . . . In other words, being born naturally, at the proper time, is a developmental need, just like walking. When that need is deprived or hindered, profound and permanent changes occur.

Mothers of cesarean babies should take these concerns into account. If cesarean-delivered babies have in fact been deprived, they will require more cuddling, skin contact, and light massage than normally delivered babies. If your baby shows any of the signs of deprivation, respond to him or her wholeheartedly.

POSSIBLE PSYCHOLOGICAL EFFECTS ON THE MOTHER

"I blamed myself for not doing my preparation exercises right," one mother told me. "I felt I had let my husband down because, after taking the class and all, he couldn't be there," said another. But a third, whose doctor planned beforehand for her husband's presence and who encouraged him to hold her hand throughout and to bathe the baby afterward, reported, "It was a wonderful experience."

Cesarean delivery need not be a psychological trauma, even if your husband cannot be present. One woman reported, "The nurse was wonderful. She talked to me all the way through. The doctors were kidding

around at first, but I told them to 'lay off,' and then they were very supportive."

Unfortunately, many women find cesarean birth an upsetting emotional experience. Nurse-author Ruth Allen reports, "A helpless feeling
is common, and afterward, a diminished self-image." Emotionally, many
women feel traumatized by the surgery and depressed afterward.
They're disappointed in themselves, assuming the blame for not being
able to have a normal delivery. She suggests reassuring the mother by
giving her the baby to hold in her arms right after birth and allowing
prepared fathers to be present during surgery. "Cesarean birth can be a
joyous experience if the mother, her husband, and her friends and relatives all are well prepared."

PREPARING FOR A GOOD CESAREAN
BIRTH EXPERIENCE

Because C-sections are becoming so common, many childbirth teachers
today routinely talk about the operation, describe preparatory and postpartum exercises, and help couples plan for an optimal arrangement in
the hospital.

If you are preparing on your own, there are three major areas to look
into:

1. At the time of this writing, estimates are that 15 percent of hospitals are reversing a long-standing prohibition and now routinely allow
fathers into the operating room so C-sections can be a family event. At
the start of the procedure, the father sits at the head of the table, by the
anesthetist, and an obstetrics nurse fills him in on what's happening.
Once the incision has been made, the screen that shields both parents
from the operating field is removed so they can watch the infant's birth.

Studies have shown that concerns about infection, that fathers will
faint or interfere, and that malpractice suits will increase all have proved
unwarranted. It should therefore become easier to arrange for your
husband's presence at the hospital of your choice. Now that medical
authorities are less concerned about projected disadvantages, they are
more willing to go along with the thinking expressed by Ruth Allen: "For
most women, the presence of the father is emotionally invaluable."

2. If you know you will be having a cesarean birth, arrange to see a
movie about one through your local C-sec group (see below) or through

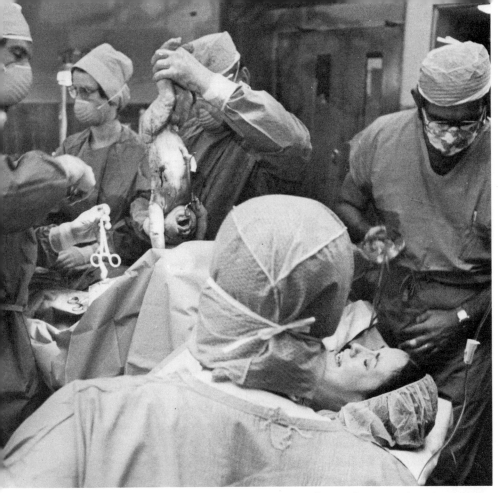

Awake and aware during Cesarean birth! (From the film: Cesarean Childbirth, *Jay Hathaway Productions, courtesy American Academy of Husband-Coached Childbirth)*

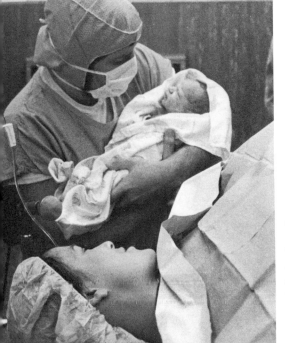

Safe in daddy's arms immediately after Cesarean birth. (From the film: Cesarean Childbirth, *Jay Hathaway Productions, courtesy American Academy of Husband-Coached Childbirth)*

your local ICEA group (see Appendix I). The first viewing will make you queasy, the second won't seem so bad, and by the third you will be raring to be the star yourself. Also speak to other women who have had cesareans. You can meet them at the C-sec meeting or by asking your doctor for the names and telephone numbers of some patients who have had them. Read about cesarean birth in the special books recommended in the Bibliography. Ask your doctor every question you can think of. The more you know about what will be happening, the better you will feel.

3. Prepare physically for your cesarean during pregnancy, and exercise afterward to recuperate. You will need to begin your exercises in bed after the operation. The exercises below are recommended to prepare your body beforehand and to help you recover safely and more easily. They will not harm your incision and are essential to stimulate healing. Exercise will help the edges of the incision come together. Even though you will not have a vaginal delivery, you should do the pelvic floor exercises in chapter 2 all during pregnancy to support the uterus and help restore the muscles afterward.

Here are the exercises to help you prepare for and recuperate after cesarean surgery. As you do them, you will find the encouragement and support of your nurse and husband very helpful.

Cesarean Preparatory Exercises

To be done in sequence.
Position: Lie or sit, well supported by pillows.

1. Diaphragmatic breathing. Place hands on V of ribs (underneath rib cage). Breathe in deeply through nose, feeling V spread apart as the diaphragm pushes down. Blow out through mouth, tightening abdominal muscles. Repeat 8 times.

2. Coughing. Make believe you're holding the two sides of your incision together (vertically if you're having a "midline incision," horizontally if you're having a "bikini cut"—ask your doctor which one it will be). Cough hard. This strengthens your diaphragm and will make it easier to cough after surgery if you have general anesthesia and secretion to spit out. (Always spit out into a tissue, never swallow secretions.)

3. Huffing. In case coughing is too difficult after surgery, practice huffing. Breathe in deeply and sharply. Force the air out while saying "Ha."

4. Flexing. Move feet up and down, at ankle joint, keeping legs straight and knees pointing up. Repeat 20 times.

5. Chest breathing. Place hands at the sides of your breasts. Breathe in and feel your chest expanding out toward hands. Blow out, 8 times.

6. Repeat coughing and huffing.

7. Pressing. Tighten thighs by pushing knees down toward the floor and squeeze buttocks together. Release. Repeat *contractions* 10 times.

8. Left chest expansion. Lie on your right side, place left hand on the left side of your chest. Breathe in deeply, moving the left side of your chest upward. Blow out, tightening abdominal muscles. Repeat 8 times.

9. Bicycle. Bend first one knee, then straighten it and bend the other. Repeat slowly 20 times.

10. Right chest expansion. Lie on your left side, place right hand on right side of chest, moving it upward with your chest as you breathe in. Blow out, pulling in abdominal muscles. Repeat 8 times.

11. More coughing and huffing.

12. Ankle rotation. Part your legs slightly, rotate ankles clockwise 15 times, and counterclockwise 15 times more.

13. Bridging. Lie down. Bend knees, feet flat on floor. Lift buttocks into the air. (This prepares you to use the bedpan after surgery.)

Cesarean Rehabilitation Exercises

Immediately after the C-section, it's important that you do some of the exercises while the anesthesia is still working so they will be less painful. With the help of your husband or nurse, do the following:

Day One

1. Diaphragmatic breathing.

2. Coughing and huffing (only necessary if you have general anesthetic).

3. Feet up and down.

4. Side of the chest breathing.

5. Coughing and huffing.

6. Tighten thighs.

Do these exercises every 2 to 3 hours, and you'll be well on your way to recovery. They will *not* stress your stitches.

Day Two

Once the doctor is satisfied that your blood pressure is stable, you will be allowed to get up and walk a short distance.

To get up, bend your knees up, roll over onto your side, and push yourself up by your arms. At the same time, slide your legs over the edge of the bed. (At least one person should be there to assist you.) Swing your feet up and down, straightening first one leg and then the other, so you won't feel faint when you get up from blood pooling in the legs.

Stand up perfectly straight; *don't* crouch in to favor the incision or recuperation will be much more uncomfortable later. Literally march around the room, heel-toe action, trying to swing your arms. Afterward, you may be allowed to sit in a chair and will feel much better. Take as many walks as you are allowed.

To the exercises of Day One, add exercises 8 through 12 from Cesarean Preparatory Exercises and do pelvic floor exercises (chapter 2).

Day Three

Add breast muscle exercise and pelvic rock from Prepartum Fitness Exercises (chapter 2).

Day Four

Pull in your abdominal muscles tightly, hold 5 seconds, then let go. Do pelvic rock while standing.

Note:

1. No heavy lifting for at least 3 weeks after delivery.
2. Gas in the intestines may be troublesome on the 2nd and 3rd day postpartum. To eliminate gas, lie on your left side and gently knead your stomach to help gas expel naturally.
3. If you need to cough, sneeze, pass a stool, laugh, etc., hold your hands flat and firm against each side of your abdomen.
4. It's easier to sit on a bedpan than lie down on top of it.
5. Nursing? It may take as long as 10 days for your milk to come in, because of the anesthesia. But it will. (Read chapter 12.)
6. Once Cesarean Rehabilitation Exercises are painless, you can proceed to regular Postpartum Exercises (chapter 2).

CESAREAN CHILDBIRTH SELF-HELP GROUPS

If you have a cesarean, you will find that afterward people will say such tactless things as "You got off easy" or "You flunked." Many people will not realize how weak and uncomfortable you feel, how long it takes to recuperate completely from this operation. You may also find it hard to hold and feed the baby. For these reasons, you will be grateful for all the advice and emotional support you can get from more experienced cesarean mothers.

You may be concerned about the future. Should you have a cesarean section next time? One woman told me, "I always thought I wanted natural childbirth until I had a cesarean. Now I feel lucky I will never have to have a labor pain." This is the kind of issue you will want to discuss with other women, and with qualified experts, invited by C. B. A. or other cesarean childbirth associations at their meetings. Sharing experiences also helps women to heal emotionally. If your husband wasn't present at your first cesarean birth, you may want to know how to arrange to have him there the next time.

Nancy Lee Krauter, who founded the Cesarean Birth Association group after the birth of her cesarean baby, describes how the organization operates: "We promote dissemination of information to parents and health professionals, and freedom of choice for every couple to have the kind of birth experience that suits their individual needs. We have helped develop model programs in several New York hospitals that include having specially prepared fathers present for the birth as well as all other family-centered practices. We offer in-service programs for health professionals and also have educational seminars for the medical and the lay community. We have meetings at which we share feelings, experiences, and options. At first, we all tend to say we feel fine, but, in fact, depression is not uncommon after a cesarean, and so are feelings of emotional loss."

To minimize unhappy feelings afterward, cesarean groups invite couples to join them and become informed before delivery, whenever possible.

Self-help groups: To find one of the growing number of C-sec support groups write to either: The Cesarean Birth Association, 125 North 12th Street, New Hyde Park, New York 10040; or C-Sec International, 15 Maynard Road, Dedham, Massachusetts 02026.

ANESTHESIA AND CESAREAN SECTION

A concern, with any childbirth medication, is the effect it may have on the baby. Epidural anesthesia, a regional block that permits the mother to remain awake during surgery and has less serious effect on the baby than a general anesthetic, is used today for most C-sections. The epidural procedure and anesthetic effects on the mother and baby are discussed in the next chapter.

6

The Pros and Cons of Childbirth Drugs

Should you or shouldn't you try for a childbirth without drugs? Can you or can't you handle the stress and possible pain? How important is it that you try?

Unlike most countries, the United States doesn't maintain a registry on drugs released for clinical use in childbirth. No one knows the full extent of drug use and the number and types of adverse reactions in patients for whom drugs are being prescribed. Yet it is conservatively estimated that more than 90 percent of mothers are given some kind of relief through medication or anesthesia in childbirth.

Most of these mothers suspect it would be better not to take any drugs and wish it were possible to do without them. They believe, however, (as do most doctors), that some kind of pain relief is usually necessary to make labor and delivery tolerable. Most doctors feel they can contain potential risks by judicious use of drugs, suggest studies showing that some drugs actually benefit the baby, and maintain that the reduction of apprehension and fear in the mother outweighs the risks of using drugs.

There are four major types of childbirth drugs. Tranquilizers are given to reduce anxiety, and analgesics decrease the pain by raising the pain threshold. General anesthesia makes the mother unconscious during birth, whereas regional anesthesia creates a temporary loss of sensation in the birthing area while the patient remains awake.

BRIEF HISTORY OF CHILDBIRTH DRUGS

Historically, painkillers have been avidly sought in every culture for use in childbirth and were used heavily until the present. "Now the pendulum is swinging from an era of excessive use toward one of minimal medication," says Dr. Stanley James.

Ether, then chloroform, were the first anesthetics used, starting in 1847. There were clerical and medical objections to interfering with God's will and the natural process, respectively, but when Queen Victoria, the secular head of the Church of England, allowed herself to be chloroformed in 1853 and again in 1857, ministerial objections were stifled.

From the start, questions about the safety and necessity of anesthesia were raised by the medical profession both in England and in the United States. Nevertheless, chloroform was commonly used until well into the twentieth century because of its ease of administration and rapid action. Very little attention was paid to the infant's reaction, except for some casual observation. It was assumed that no matter how poor the infant's initial state, as long as he ultimately appeared normal, then he had suffered only transient difficulties. Only in the last decade have experts (primarily developmental psychologists) begun to question whether there might be any long-term detrimental effects on the baby.

Twilight sleep (morphine and scopolamine) was first tried in 1902 and within a short time was used extensively. It was relatively safe for the mothers, but produced severely depressed babies. Barbiturates were first reported in 1924, used in combination with other drugs. However, some doctors observed that heavy medication was associated with prolonged labor and stillbirth.

Regional anesthesia became prominent in the 1940s and is presently the most popular means of eliminating the pain of childbirth. Also in the 1940s, the English doctor, Grantly Dick-Read, toured the United States and presented his natural-childbirth method of education and support, which stressed that labor is a natural process. Although many doctors continued to use drugs, his work made many obstetricians more conscious of the need to secure the full cooperation of patients, "making the psychologic management of the patient an indispensable basic sedative," according to Dr. James. It was Grantly Dick-Read's work, in Dr. James's opinion, that paved the way for smaller doses of medication.

The belief that the natural-childbirth movement has decreased overall drug use is challenged by some drug experts, like developmental psychologist Dr. Yvonne Brackbill of the University of Florida. Citing recent studies and statistics that indicate that drug intake has been increasing in the last few years, she says, "Some drugs are used less, but some, like oxytocin, are markedly more common." Still, medication is no longer seen as a panacea.

"There has been a dramatic reduction in both infant and maternal mortality in the last fifty years," Dr. James points out. "As a result, mothers are not afraid of dying in childbirth. Improvement in the mental attitude of mothers has been a major factor in reducing their demands for medication."

While few women today are afraid of dying or becoming seriously ill because of pregnancy or childbirth, many are still quite apprehensive about the experience, which has become increasingly unfamiliar as our society has changed. Ignorance about childbirth is one reason for continued reliance on drugs; the other is the belief of most obstetricians that there is sufficient pain in normal childbirth to require the use of drugs or anesthetics. They would agree with Dr. Finster's assessment: "A well-prepared woman might well choose some form of pain relief if her labor is more difficult than the average."

With the easy accessibility of drugs and ready encouragement to use them, without a tradition of drug-free childbirth to back her up in a frightening situation, the average American woman still asks for and receives drug relief in childbirth.

ADVANTAGES AND DISADVANTAGES OF DRUGS

Great controversy rages over the value and/or harm of using drugs in childbirth. On the one hand, experts are sure they are administering drugs without harming mothers and babies and cite research findings indicating the advantages of drugs. On the other hand, natural-childbirth advocates are convinced that every drug is disadvantageous in normal childbirth, for mother and baby, and cite medical studies to support their claim. Experts on both sides question the others' findings, pointing to flaws in research methods, and present strong arguments to support their views. Because much of the research necessarily has been done on animals, it is particularly difficult to make an objective evaluation. As has been pointed out, it is the mother's state of mind and informational preparation, as well as her physiological response, that determines her need for drugs in normal childbirth. The final decision needs to be made by the informed consumer.

Drs. James and Finster of Columbia University's College of Physicians and Surgeons are medical experts who have done considerable research with drugs. They feel that the public is both overlooking the advantages of drugs and overestimating their disadvantages.

Dr. James, who has been involved in barbiturate research, makes a case for using these drugs: "Barbiturates can lower the requirements for oxygen to the fetal brain and prevent brain damage. Research indicates that barbiturates can also be used when a baby must be induced prematurely to speed up the development of liver enzymes, to prevent jaundice. Other drugs [hormones] can accelerate the maturation of the premature fetal lung and lead to the prevention of breathing difficulties at birth. Our knowledge of fetal pharmacology is in its infancy. We need more information, but we already know there are advantages as well as disadvantages to using drugs. Although analgesic agents may prolong labor and indirectly exert a harmful effect on the fetus, certain drugs can also have value for the well-being of the baby. Maternal anxiety can be a hazard. It can reduce uterine blood flow and the course of labor. It can cause overbreathing, which results in too low a level of carbon dioxide, leading to lowering of the maternal blood pressure and deficient blood flow to the placenta and a low oxygen level for the baby. If labor is 'tumultuous,' with overly rapid and strong contractions, sedating the mother to slow labor down can be very important to avoid asphyxiating the baby, since the blood flow to the placenta ceases during very strong uterine contractions. A variety of drugs can calm the central nervous system and relieve pain. If these are given in small enough doses, they will reach the baby but not harm him."

Dr. Finster adds, "There is no evidence whatever that a judicious amount of drugs has an adverse effect on the baby. Drugs are good, bad, or indifferent depending on when and how much is given and under what circumstances. . . . Fetal circulation protects the fetal brain from the immediate effects of drugs administered to the mother. Drugs go into the fetus in less than a minute, but the fetal liver removes a lot, and then there is rapid dilution within the fetal circulation. If a drug leaves the mother's blood rapidly, it never builds up in the fetus's brain. We anesthetize the *mother*, not the baby. However, if large amounts of drugs are administered repeatedly to the mother or if she is maintained under prolonged general anesthesia, these protective mechanisms are no longer effective and the baby is born depressed."

Medical sociologist Doris Haire has been a leader in the fight against the widespread use of drugs in normal childbirth. She argues against the applicability of much of the animal research referred to and reports other studies, with different outcomes: "It is misleading to imply that only large amounts of obstetric drugs have an adverse effect on the fetus and newborn infant. A study by J.C. Morrison of the University of Tennessee, published in 1976, has shown that only 50 milligrams of Demerol—which is considered a small dose—caused mild depression in one out of four infants in a group of eighty births, depending on how rapidly it was metabolized by the mother. While there are drugs that can alter the symptoms of this newborn depression, there is no guarantee that such drugs prevent long-term neurologic damage. Far too many babies are requiring oxygen immediately after birth! Although many doctors feel this can be given with no ill effect, there are research findings that the onset of respiration and sucking is less prompt in anesthetized babies, that they frequently are irritable and have impaired motor control, which may or may not be temporary."

While there are heated arguments about how many babies are born depressed, whether or not this is due to drugs or other events during childbirth, whether research done with wild monkeys is valid when applied to humans, and the like, the fundamental dispute between the traditionalists and the natural-childbirth advocates is over the question of whether drugs and anesthetics have long-range effects on the baby's brain and neurological system. Doctors who use anesthesia believe that adverse effects wear off within days, and that there are no long-range deleterious effects on the baby's brain, its future development, or its learning capacity. Natural-childbirth advocates counter with the research and current work of Dr. Yvonne Brackbill of the University of Florida, which points to permanent structure and functional changes from childbirth drugs. In her article "Obstetrical Medication and Infant Behavior," she says:

> The newborn human baby is an organism poorly positioned to deal with toxic agents. Drugs enter the central nervous system readily because of incomplete blood/brain barriers; they lodge

in brain structures that are still developing and therefore at high risk to damage; they cannot readily be transformed into nontoxic compounds since the necessary liver functions are immature, and they cannot readily be excreted because of inefficient kidney function.

Dr. Brackbill cites circumstantial evidence that often it is not mothers' preferences or requests but rather doctors' and hospitals' administrative practices that determine whether a mother receives drugs and which ones she is given. Some doctors habitually use epidural anesthesia, others general anesthetics. She points out that "standing orders" for Nembutol, Demerol, and the like are widespread, that "the more a patient is treated according to a standing order, which allows nurses and pharmacists to dispense medication in a physician's absence, the less voice a patient has in decision making about her own medication."

PUBLIC COMPLACENCY ABOUT DRUGS

Dr. Brackbill's findings of long-term neurological damage are shocking because most of us complacently believe that so long as our Food and Drug Administration does not ban the use of a drug, it must be safe. Says Doris Haire, "The FDA does not guarantee the safety of *any* drug. It has no specific designation for 'safe.' Many drugs presently given have never been officially reviewed, released, or approved for use by the FDA. Before 1962, in fact, the FDA had no power to approve a drug as safe for use or marketing, and the vast majority of drugs for pregnant women were on the market before 1962. Once a drug is on the market, it is rarely taken off."

There is no regulation that requires drug manufacturers to alert consumers to the consequences—indirect and direct—of using their drugs. As Doris Haire says, "Drugs used to induce labor may precipitate the need for other measures that can be traumatic to the baby. Epidural anesthesia, now being touted as the 'Cadillac' of regional anesthesias, is an example of complicated consequences. When we choose epidural, we also choose a great number of medical procedures such as forceps that are needed to increase the safety of the method."

Epidurals, now the most popular form of regional anesthesia, require a great deal of skill in administering according to Dr. Michael Bergman. Before planning delivery with epidural anesthesia, a mother should

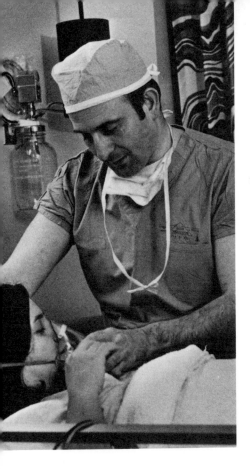

It is important to ascertain whether the benefits of anesthesia outweigh the risks in your situation. (From the Parenting Pictures film: The Cesarean Birth Experience, *Courter Films and Associates)*

At Englewood Hospital in New Jersey, a husband supports his wife as the anesthesiologist administers an epidural. The mother remains awake, but feels nothing from the breasts down. (Alison Ehrlich Wachstein, from Pregnant Moments, *Morgan & Morgan, 1978)*

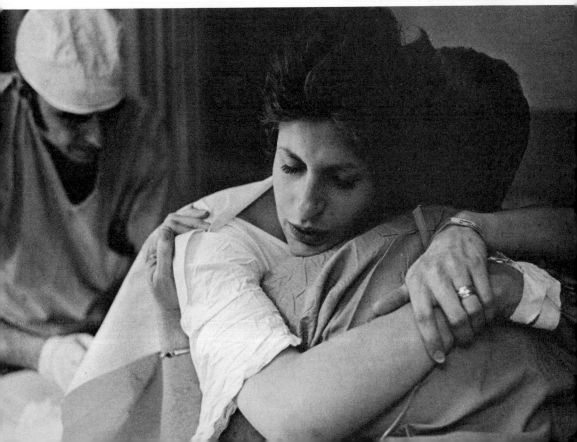

know that "the needle must be properly introduced into the outer space around the spinal column. If a mistake is made, the large amount of drug used—twenty-five times that given in direct spinal injection—can cause paralysis, shock, or even death of the mother, and affect the baby's heart and oxygen supply. There are dangers with all anesthesia, but they are not reportable complications and don't appear in statistics or research unless the patient dies."

WHAT IS YOUR POINT OF VIEW?

Now that you know the possible hazards of using drugs in childbirth, you may be determined to have a drug-free childbirth, if at all possible. Unfortunately, you're likely to feel like an oddball since such a large proportion of mothers *do* take drugs, and you may be worried about whether or not you are competent to make such a decision and capable of carrying it through. Or you may be afraid that you cannot predict how you will behave when the time comes. There are a number of things you can do to prepare yourself emotionally for natural childbirth. The most important is to deal with your ignorance and fears now so you won't have to cope with them during delivery.

1. *Desensitize yourself to childbirth.* The best way to master apprehension is not by putting it out of your mind or offering yourself false reassurances. It is, rather, to become as familiar with labor and delivery as you possibly can beforehand. One excellent way is by watching documentary movies about childbirth. There are occasional television specials that show childbirth more or less explicitly, and some are excellent. Lamaze and Bradley groups have childbirth films showing their own methods. They can be seen at meetings open to the public, with discussion afterward. The ICEA (see part three) also has a film and record directory. It can tell you where and how to rent films inexpensively for a small group of your own.

You can expect to become quite agitated the first time you watch any childbirth movie. The suspense is terrific, even though you know how the story turns out. Seeing the blood, hearing the sounds, is part of the desensitization. After a few movies, you will find that your apprehension about your own delivery is turning to excited anticipation. That's the point.

2. *Talk to new mothers.* Women in childbirth education classes and

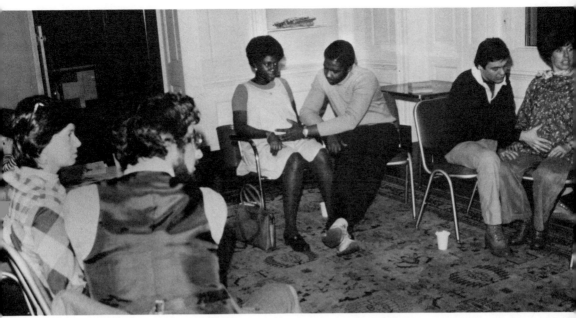

The childbirth education class is the place to air concerns and share experiences. (Mariette Pathy Allen/Maternity Center Association)

postpartum groups of every kind are willing, even eager, to talk about their experiences and feelings during childbirth. The ICEA person in your own area (see Appendix I) can direct you to these local groups. You may feel freer to ask candid questions of sympathetic strangers than of friends, relatives, or acquaintances.

Ask the women what hurt them most. Ask if they were medicated and how it felt. Ask if medication helped, and how they felt about using it afterward. How did they know when to ask for drugs?

Was it possible for any women to relax without drugs in childbirth? How did they do it? What helped—preparatory exercises, breathing, mind control, their husbands' presence, the reassurance of the doctor and nurse? Did any of them lose control unexpectedly? What happened then?

Ask about everything that concerns *you*. You may be surprised at some of the answers. Some women will tell you how much they regretted what they did—whatever it was. Others are pleased as punch with whatever happened. One woman, who had planned for a natural childbirth and ended up with an emergency cesarean, told me, "It was a fabulous experience. I'm glad I'll be having my next baby by cesarean, especially after hearing the other women yell." Another explains why she likes to talk about her childbirths: "Even in the one childbirth that wasn't good there were terrific moments, which I like to relive—the physical feelings of my baby emerging from my body. It was a wonderful experience."

In my own survey of new mothers, I was impressed by how often childbirth education and hospital personnel support were mentioned as the most important factors: "I didn't end up with natural childbirth, but what I learned about what to expect was priceless." Or: "The nurses paid more attention to one another than to me, except to tell me not to move. My husband felt he was in the way. At one point, in transition, I just yelled and refused to push, until the doctor applied abdominal pressure and brought me back to reality."

The worst memories were about lack of communication, not knowing what was happening: "In the recovery room, I hemorrhaged, and they wouldn't tell me what was happening. They sent my husband out, and he was waiting for me upstairs for three hours."

Some women will tell you proudly that they never lost control for a minute, and why. "The doctor was there, my husband was there, right by my side." Others report that losing control was the part of the experience that was most meaningful for them. "Once I let myself cry, everyone was wonderful. I felt cared about and supported all the way through."

A small group of women will tell you that maintaining self-control was never an issue that crossed their minds. They felt entitled to have a full experience in their own way. They were able to be completely spontaneous and involved. Many women report, "It was the most wonderful experience of my life." One said, "I feel my childbirths can happen only a few times, and I want to enjoy them to the fullest. These are the experiences that most belong to me."

From your discussions with new mothers you will be able to pinpoint the personal qualities and attitudes about childbirth that make for success or lack of success in the natural method. Then you can begin to develop those parts of yourself that will be assets and downplay your negative tendencies, getting yourself into the proper frame of mind for a full and happy adventure of your own.

3. *Arrange for supportive coaching.* Natural-childbirth educators call it "verbal anesthesia," and doctors feel it is "the indispensable basic sedative." In the last ten years, American obstetrics has swung fully behind the concept of having a loving, supportive companion through labor and delivery. Approximately 60 percent of fathers now see their babies delivered, compared to less than 5 percent a decade ago. No longer does a woman have to be afraid of being alone in a new and

frightening situation. Everyone needs strong emotional support under stress. By accepting that need, and arranging for a companion in delivery to coach and support you, you are taking the first—and probably the most important—step toward having a successful drug-free childbirth.

Be honest about who makes you feel most comfortable and secure. It's important to follow your feelings, as well as your husband's. Discuss it candidly. If he's queasy about being present and you'd really rather have your mother there, have her. In most hospitals, you're allowed just one companion, though in the more family-centered situations, a mother can surround herself with as much support as she desires. Arrange for what will be most helpful to you personally—handholding, jokes, a kiss, backrubs, etc. You will be center stage, getting all the consideration and attention. Make the most of it!

4. *Talk it over with your doctor.* Discuss with him what drugs he generally uses. Ask him to let you read the "package inserts." Tell him your feelings, fears, and reservations. It's important to find a doctor whose attitudes about drugs and anethesia fit easily with your own. If he usually uses epidurals and is going along with drug-free, natural childbirth only to accommodate you, he will not have the conviction and enthusiasm, or the firsthand experience, of the doctor who usually attends drug-free births. But if you communicate, his conviction about a particular drug or anesthetic may convince you that it would be good for you. Discussion is the best way to develop full confidence and peace of mind about choices. You might ask the doctor for permission to use his name at the local medical library. Read about the planned anesthesia in advance. The medical librarian will help you find the studies.

With that kind of easy communication and full preparation, you will find yourself able to discuss drugs during your labor, knowledgeably and confidently. You will know when to ask for pain relief, without feeling unsure or disappointed in yourself afterward.

Emotional support and approval of your goals by medical attendants as well as your companion is probably the most strengthening ingredient for a successful natural childbirth.

7

The Natural Way

By now you are aware that "managed and monitored" childbirth has many complications and drawbacks. Although you will be "out of it" briefly, you may be "stuck with it" afterward. Many women are selecting natural childbirth, not because they relish the experience but because being awake and aware seems the safer route for the baby and themselves.

There are many different motivations for undertaking natural childbirth, and many degrees of commitment. You needn't belong to any one school of thought or have any one particular personality type to succeed in natural childbirth. Methods of preparation have been designed to match different philosophies and temperaments. They are available nationwide, and you should be able to find a course that will prepare you for your own best way.

This chapter will tell you about many of these methods, how to match yourself up with one of them, and how to locate the right class in your community. A good book that explains each method in detail will be recommended so you will be able to read all about it before making a final choice.

WHY PREPARE?

"If it's all so natural, then why do I have to prepare for the experience?" you may be thinking. Theoretically, you don't have to. If you have no fear of labor or the hospital, if you already know how to relax under stress, if you are informed about the physiology of labor and familiar with delivery-room procedures, you may not need to enroll for any classes. But if you feel it would be useful and strengthening to learn about the various ways to deliver without medication, if you want to learn more about the advantages to the baby and yourself of a natural childbirth under normal circumstances, if you want the opportunity to ask questions and discuss all your concerns with an expert, the chances are you will decide to enroll for help.

THE MATERNITY CENTER ASSOCIATION

Because of their special role in childbirth education and in improving maternal and child health care in the United States, I would like to tell you about the outstanding contributions of the Maternity Center Association, which began as a small group of concerned women in New York City. Prepared childbirth really started with the Maternity Center Association. This was the group that invited Grantly Dick-Read to America from England to teach his method. They incorporated his ideas into their preparatory childbirth courses. They have also been in the forefront in bringing childbirth education and prenatal care to poor people, developing a large, safe home-birth service by nurse-midwives that has performed with excellent mortality and morbidity statistics for many years, and training nurse-midwives. Now they are testing the concept of "homelike delivery" in a childbearing center located in their townhouse-office in a lovely old section of Manhattan. The Maternity Center Association is a unique voluntary organization that for sixty years has pioneered advances in childbirth.

The association's goal is that "every baby born will be a welcomed baby and have the high quality of care needed before, during and after birth." When it began, America had the highest maternal death rate of the developed nations in the world. Now it has one of the lowest, and the association had a great deal to do with that progress.

The Maternity Center Association has focused on new and different projects according to the needs of the time. In the 1930s, its greatest contribution was in nurse-midwifery training. It started the first training school, and students delivered a substantial number of babies in poor areas of New York until the home-birth service closed in 1958, due to the deterioration of the inner city. Most of the graduate midwives went on to deliver skilled care, under the direction of obstetricians, in isolated rural communities all over America. The association meanwhile continued its childbirth preparation classes, and middle-class New Yorkers began to reach out for its services. Maternity Center Association books, posters, and education materials are used in childbirth classes and community projects all over the United States.

It was in the 1940s that the association sponsored visits from Dr. Grantly Dick-Read and Helen Heardman, leading exponents of natural childbirth in England. Maternity Center incorporated some of their ideas and techniques into its classes, developing the Dick-Read/Maternity Center method. Meanwhile, its home delivery and nurse-midwifery training programs continued to grow and flourish, and other communities asked for help in establishing programs.

The focus of the fifties was on helping the natural movements to develop and sponsoring nurse-midwifery training programs in other parts of the United States.

Every Maternity Center Association program was considered innovative, even questionable, when it started. Yet each one has enriched the childbirth experience of Americans.

The Maternity Center Association remains the place to call for a referral if you want: a Leboyer doctor, a family-centered hospital with rooming-in, a natural-childbirth doctor, or just a good class in natural childbirth.

THE DICK-READ/MATERNITY CENTER METHOD OF NATURAL CHILDBIRTH

These are the classes in the Dick-Read Natural Childbirth method first developed by Grantly Dick-Read's *Childbirth Without Fear* (see Bibliography). In the 1940s, with this book and extensive public lecturing, Dick-Read introduced the concept of natural childbirth to the United States, and many believe that his original method is still the best.

However, most "Dick-Read courses" are modifications of the original method. With a few exceptions, such as the Gamper classes offered in the Midwest, natural-childbirth courses today teach Lamaze or shallow, panting breathing rather than the deep, relaxed abdominal breathing recommended by Dick-Read. Most women find it easier to learn the Lamaze exercises and to use the breathing to deflect attention from their bodily sensations than to concentrate on their bodies, which is necessary in abdominal breathing. The Bradley approach (described later) still uses the abdominal-breathing method, but classes in Dick-Read natural childbirth today are really a combination of the old and the new.

Today husbands are included in Dick-Read classes, just as they are in Lamaze or Bradley, even though this practice was unknown when Dick-Read introduced his method. Their inclusion is a logical extension of Dick-Read's ideas for providing emotional support to the mother, and nurse Jayne Wiggins of Long Island, New York, who has been teaching the Dick-Read method since classes were first developed at the Maternity Center Association, says, "The emotional support of a loving companion now is the most important component of the method."

Basically, the philosophy remains the same—eliminate destructive fear, tension, and resultant pain through proper education and sufficient emotional support. The course not only conditions you to cope with tension (like Lamaze), but emphasizes the information that will allay fear and prevent tension. This includes: exercises (breathing control, relaxation of muscles), information (what to expect in a normal situation, what the mother can do to help herself, what she can expect from others), and support (guidance, direction, reassurance, and empathy).

Dick-Read's natural childbirth is as much concerned with preparation for parenthood as with childbirth itself. Usually, every maternity patient in a hospital that offers a course can take it whether or not she intends to have natural childbirth. Hospitals especially encourage high-risk teen-agers to come to the classes, since the nutritional information helps reduce their incidence of toxemia and the labor and delivery information helps allay their fears. It has been found that high-risk patients who cannot have natural childbirth nonetheless do better than they otherwise would in labor and delivery if they have taken the natural-childbirth course.

My objection to these courses is essentially the same as my objection to the Lamaze courses:—they aren't problem-centered enough. They gloss over possible complications and abnormalities unless someone specifically asks about them. In my view, that is not thorough preparation, particularly with the rising rate of C-sections and the frequency with which breech position and other deviations from normality occur. Obviously, many natural-childbirth teachers don't agree with my point of view, although there has been a shift generally in the direction of discussing possible problems that might arise in labor and delivery. These teachers maintain (shortsightedly, I think) that their students are

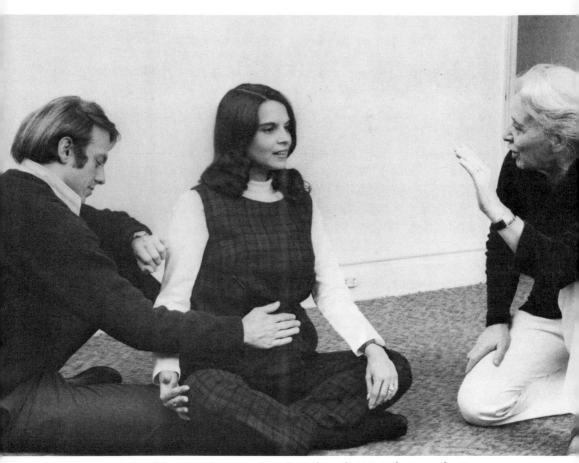

Elisabeth Bing, renowned co-founder of ASPO, has taught Lamaze method to thousands of couples. (Erika Stone)

coming to learn about the *normal*, natural process, not deviations; that they have too much material to cover in the limited number of sessions to add more about complications and abnormalities; and that too much discussion of abnormal possibilities would upset parents-to-be.

As a psychotherapist, I have learned that people do not worry about problems they hear about unless they're already concerned and anxious. The best way to clear away anxieties is to explore feelings fully. As nurse-educator Ruth Allen observes, "There should be no obstetrical secrets. Women envision far worse in their imaginations."

LAMAZE PREPARED CHILDBIRTH

By far the most popular natural-childbirth method in America today is Lamaze prepared childbirth, named for the French doctor who developed the method. It seems well suited to the American character, which values teamwork, partnership, rationality, and taking responsibility.

Lamaze courses are the easiest to find in most communities. They combine physical, mental, emotional, and informational preparation for a woman and the companion of her choice, usually her husband. The Lamaze method relies heavily on physical and psychological conditioning.

Here is the Lamaze point of view, as expressed by Lamaze educator Valmai Elkins: "Almost every woman can experience childbirth as a normal but extremely strenuous activity similar to an athletic event; like any athletic activity, it requires dedicated preparation."

The woman conditions her body throughout pregnancy with special exercises. She trains her mind to respond automatically to each type of labor contraction. For the early stages, she is taught to relax her muscles at will and to deflect her attention from the contraction through breathing (there are about thirty different patterns), gentle stomach massage, and eye-focusing. This last works much like the trick dental patients discover for themselves: Concentrate on a spot on the wall until the dentist finishes drilling.

For the later stages, the woman learns to "push on command" of her coaches—to push the baby gently through the birth canal. Throughout the delivery, she is *awake and aware* and kept informed of her progress by the doctor and nurse. She is, in fact, a cooperating and rational member of the childbirth team, which consists of four people—herself, her husband (usually), the doctor, and the nurse.

Since labor and delivery are perceived as stressful, even potentially overwhelming experiences, Lamaze conditioning is designed to teach the woman how to brake herself—physically and psychologically—in order to maintain self-control. The rationale is similar to that for teaching inexperienced skiers the snowplow right away—to give them the security of knowing they can control their speed as they ease themselves down a scary hill.

The husband is both coach and emotional support. He takes the course along with his wife, helps her at home with the conditioning exercises, and "coaches, coaxes, and comforts her" through labor and delivery. While most hospitals now permit Lamaze-prepared fathers into labor rooms, some will not allow them to accompany their wives to the

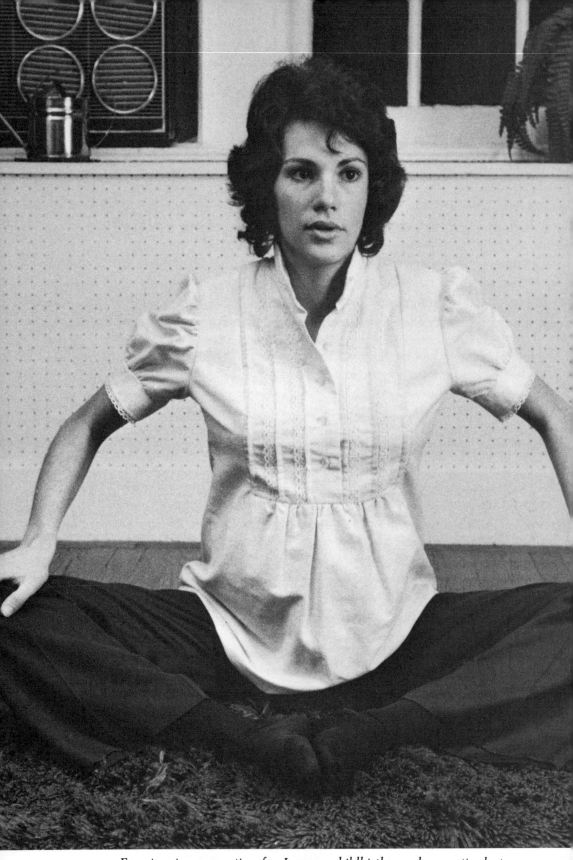

Exercises in preparation for Lamaze childbirth can be practiced at home as well as in classes.(Erika Stone)

delivery room, or will ask them to leave if heavy medication or anesthesia is required. If you want another "companion of choice," you'll have to stipulate this beforehand. The coach is kept fully informed, along with the mother, and participates with her and the doctor in decisions about using obstetric interventions, drugs, or anesthesia.

The Lamaze method is popular in this country because Americans value self-control, mastery of experience, and acceptance of the doctor's authority. Lamaze training gives a woman the tools she needs to succeed in the most socially acceptable manner possible. She is kept fully occupied with exercises and breathing, so she isn't likely to be overwhelmed by her feelings. She learns to distract herself from the physical sensations rather than become engulfed by them. She is expected to behave as a rational adult at all times.

Unfortunately, rationality is overesteemed in our culture. Many women ask for painkillers, even anesthesia, so they can continue to behave in the approved rational way, which bolsters their self-image of being grown-up and sensible. In my view, a little less emphasis on self-control and a little more expression of real feelings wouldn't hurt the childbirth situation a bit. However, if you tend to be a sensible, conforming, brave person—and you like yourself that way—a Lamaze delivery is a definite possibility. Many women do feel more comfortable with this kind of prepared childbirth than with any other. For a later delivery, when you're more experienced and self-confident and less concerned with others' opinion of you, a more permissive method and a freer atmosphere may be your choice.

The greatest drawback of the Lamaze method is its equation of a normal, uneventful childbirth with success. When difficulties arise, many women find themselves insufficiently prepared to cope with them. They feel like failures if they ask for pain relief or anesthesia, or if some surgical intervention becomes necessary.

The Lamaze doctors I spoke to were tremendously enthusiastic about the method. Without exception, they favor having prepared fathers in the delivery room. Most agree with the doctor who said, "The method is a pleasure to work with. Lamaze has a tight teacher training program. They demand good people and they deliver prepared parents."

The doctor is probably referring to the training given by the national organization of the American Society for Psycho-Prophylaxis in Obstetrics. After a rigorous course, teachers must actively participate in an

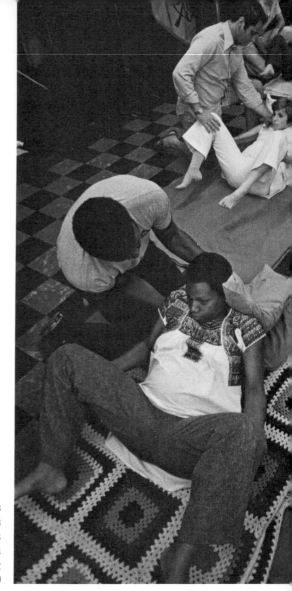

Private Lamaze classes are often smaller and more personal than hospital classes. Here mothers learn to "push" on command. (Alison Ehrlich Wachstein, from Pregnant Moments, *Morgan & Morgan, 1978)*

ongoing educational program. All professionals associated with ASPO—obstetricians as well as teachers—attend regular meetings of their own professional group plus educational meetings that are open to the interested public. That's how they keep up with new developments in the field as they are taking place.

PRIVATE ASPO–LAMAZE

Most people register for private ASPO classes in the last three months of pregnancy. It is wise to attend an open meeting earlier in pregnancy to make the contacts that will help you through the entire childbirth experience. You will be assisted in finding a good doctor and a hospital that is sympathetic to Lamaze. You will have the opportunity to meet other couples having a baby about the same time as you are, who share your ideas and values. When you attend the open meeting, you will be shown a film of a Lamaze delivery, usually *The Story of Eric.* A discussion and question-and-answer period follows.

Most private ASPO courses are six or seven weeks long, although some new pilot programs start earlier and continue right through pregnancy. Parents develop quite personal, supportive relationships with their childbirth instructors during the course, which stands them in good stead during and after the delivery. Sometimes the teacher will serve as childbirth coach (*monatrice,* the French term, is still used). More often, she will visit you in the hospital after the birth. Private classes usually cost from $30 to $50, with scholarships available as needed. Some well-known teachers do charge considerably more.

You will be referred to a number of ASPO teachers in your neighborhood; try to meet more than one before you sign up for a class. It is important that you and the teacher relate well. Most of the teachers are warmhearted and informal, but each is an individual and it's the one you relate to best who can teach and support you most.

I believe the private ASPO course is more helpful than the one given in the hospital. The hospital teacher will be an expert, but she won't be as free to work in the best tradition of consumer advocacy. Private teachers, on the other hand, will offer you a copy of the local hospital survey, if there is one, which compares the maternity facilities and policies of every hospital in your area. Teachers know the doctors personally and can describe their manner and procedures of delivery in a personal way. That is a very good way of finding resources in your community that best fit what you need.

HOSPITAL ASPO–LAMAZE

By definition, hospital classes cannot be as consumer oriented as private classes. Part of the instructor's job, as a hospital employee, is to prepare mothers to fit nicely into hospital routines and delivery procedures. A Lamaze educator at one hospital told me proudly, "Few couples who have been through our classes here in the hospital object to the rules and regulations."

It's my impression that women who take private ASPO classes are more motivated to get through childbirth without painkillers or anesthesia than those who are prepared in the hospital classes. One childbirth educator confided, "More than 50 percent of our mothers end up with epidurals. . . . I prepare mothers for a baby who is floppy and gray."

I wonder how much of this poor result is due to the subtle sabotage of having an anesthesiologist in routine attendance in natural-childbirth delivery rooms, and how much to the low expectation of success on the part of the doctors who deliver and the childbirth educators who teach at the institution. To be a success, natural childbirth requires a thoroughly relaxed and confident mother, a convinced and patient doctor, an enthusiastic coach, and a medical atmosphere that supports the natural process.

Since the cost of private and hospital classes is the same (even the teachers are often the same), since husband certifications from private classes are acceptable to hospital administrations, and since private classes get the same tour of the hospital facilities before delivery as hospital classes, I can think of no advantage to taking the ASPO course in a hospital. Hospital classes usually are much larger, too, which makes personal attention less possible. We Americans suffer from a "supermarket complex." We think that if something is purchased from a big establishment it's necessarily better. Not at all, in the case of hospital vs. private ASPO courses.

To register for classes: In Appendix II, you will find a registry of state ASPO coordinators. The one closest to you will refer you to your local chapter, which will supply you with the names and telephone numbers of teachers in your own neighborhood and local doctors who are members.

These hospital courses are offering a fine community service. Many are free, and the teachers are cordial to outsiders. Parents taking private Lamaze classes sometimes are permitted to sit in for the baby-care information. To accommodate working parents, some courses are given in the evening. Your local Board of Health or ICEA state coordinator (see Appendix I) will refer you to the closest hospital that offers the course. Some hospitals do charge about $40 for the course, so check in advance of registration.

PEP (PREPARING EXPECTANT PARENTS, INC.)

Nonmedically-trained PEP teachers are resented by some of the nurse-teachers of ASPO, who feel that recognition for Lamaze was hard won by their organization and that only professionals are qualified to teach childbirth education. Yet PEP mother-teachers also are well trained, and are subject to a yearly review by their board of directors. As mothers with unmedicated Lamaze deliveries and successful breast-feeding experience behind them, they feel fully qualified to teach other mothers. In fact, PEP courses are richer in breast-feeding information than most ASPO classes.

PEP courses begin in the third trimester. There are usually eight to ten classes, for just $25. The teachers work for nothing but expenses, and send student fees to the national office to expand the organization. This central office publishes excellent student and teacher manuals, comparable in quality to the ASPO manuals. The teachers I have met appear to be enthusiastic, determined, and dedicated. They are very involved with helping new mothers breast-feed successfully and also spend a great deal of their free time in community work. In my community, they have been very successful in improving the local hospital's family-centered program, helping to design a "birthing room" and a plan for sibling visitation.

To register for classes: Write to PEP, Box 838, Pomona, California 91769, for a directory of PEP instructors. Your ICEA coordinator (Appendix I) also will know if there is a PEP group nearby or if there is another qualified and certified mother-led group in your area.

THE BRADLEY METHOD—
HUSBAND-COACHED CHILDBIRTH

Although this method was developed almost thirty years ago by a Denver obstetrician, only now, in the decade of the "natural way," is it enthusiastically being adopted by young Americans.

The American Academy of Husband-Coached Childbirth was founded by Jay and Marge Hathaway, a young couple who were helped to deliver normally by Dr. Robert Bradley after unfortunate earlier experiences. (Jay Hathaway is also a fine documentary filmmaker, specializing in movies about childbirth.) They have been training couples in the method since 1970, and since 1972, it has been called the Bradley method.

I prefer to call it "relationship-centered childbirth" since the focus of preparation is on uniting the couple and improving their communication in preparation for childbirth. Classes are used to discuss marital stresses, sexual communication, parental roles, and nutrition as well as to prepare for labor and delivery. Relaxation exercises are demonstrated, and instructors also spend a lot of time preparing couples to cope well with hospital regulations and to improve their relationship with their doctor.

Other childbirth educators call this the "no-method" method because it doesn't attempt to teach specific exercises and breathing patterns but rather helps people find their own ways to relax. Behind the lack of formality is a lot of sound reasoning, it seems to me.

Jim and Jane Pittenger, who teach family-centered childbirth based on the Bradley method in Connecticut, explain, "We want the couple to be the center of the experience, not ourselves. Bradley is for people who can trust their bodies, who don't need an authority figure, and who find their support in the marital relationship."

Some exercises, including the pelvic floor exercises and the Kegel exercises (see chapter 2), are suggested and demonstrated. There is great emphasis on proper food in pregnancy. (Tom Brewer's film *Nutrition in Pregnancy*, which was produced by Jay Hathaway, is shown). The prospective mothers write down all the food they eat for a week, then discuss the nutritional content of their diets in class.

Abdominal breathing—deep rhythmic breaths with a relaxed belly—is the method taught in class. Husbands learn how to massage their wives from the extremities toward the heart. They observe their wives' favorite sleeping positions, which then are recommended for a most relaxed delivery.

"You need nine months to prepare yourself mentally and physically for childbirth," say David and Lee Stewart, who teach the method in Missouri. "That's why we have an early-bird class." This is an open session at which a Bradley birth film is shown and the philosophy of the couple as the center of the experience is discussed. *Happy Birth-Day* is the movie. It has a rollicking sound track, a beaming mother as the star, and the supporting cast wears jolly T-shirts—"Baby-Catcher" for the

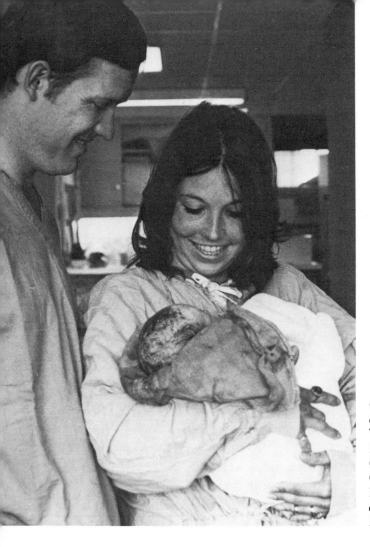

Cassie and Barry Kennedy walk out of the delivery room, after a "Bradley birth" at West Park Hospital, Canoga Park, California. (From the film: Childbirth For The Joy of It, Part II, *Jay Hathaway Productions, courtesy American Academy of Husband-Coached Childbirth)*

doctor, and "Coach" for the husband.

Parents begin with the first three of eight classes as early in pregnancy as they like. A solid foundation is provided by discussions of nutrition, relaxation exercises, and role-playing to practice communicating well with the doctor.

Here is the Pittengers' description of those early sessions: "What couples get first is a large dose of consumer advocacy. Option lists are developed, to clarify the kind of delivery they want. They role-play asking the obstetrician to arrange it. We find he's more likely to be open and receptive while you're still shopping around than once you're committed. Cooperative doctors are available. You just have to locate them."

There are six hundred trained Bradley teachers in thirty states, though not all of them are actively teaching at present. The national office will advise you if there is one in your community. The cost varies from about $34 to $50, but some teachers, like the Pittengers, will barter.

Unlike Lamaze, which helps you control the sensations of labor, Bradley encourages mothers to trust themselves, let themselves get completely involved, and enjoy the experience. The importance of this difference should not be underestimated. When a woman does not have to perform according to someone else's expectations and standards, the chances are much greater that she will find childbirth an emotionally fulfilling experience. Many of the Lamaze instructors are incorporating this freer philosophy and becoming less rigid about prescribing set exercises and breathing patterns.

If the Bradley method is available in your area, I recommend that you explore the possibilities of using it. If you're the kind of person who likes to do your own thing and can count (a great deal) on your husband to help you do it, then I recommend the Bradley method to you. It's not the techniques, it's the philosophy of Bradley that is unique. Every option—home birth, breast-feeding, early discharge from the hospital—is discussed openly and evaluated by the couple. As the Pittengers put it, "Parents who choose to participate actively in childbearing are competent to participate in the decision making."

One doctor who works frequently with Bradley couples is Dr. Ilan Israeli in New York. "I like the method," he says. "It concentrates on sensations and experiences, not on exercises. It's the same as the original Dick-Read method, except that parents feel the delivery should not divide them." Dr. Israeli, it must be said, is an exceptional doctor who likes "a lot of discussion and questions from parents. It makes my practice much more interesting." This willingness to engage in full and open communication with parents is necessary in the "baby-catcher" on the Bradley team.

Not too many readers will feel confident enough in their first pregnancy to try Bradley. More likely they will want the carefully controlled Lamaze experience, if they're willing to try natural childbirth at all. We learn about ourselves and what we want from childbirth from one delivery to the next. Because a first-time mother-to-be doesn't know how it feels to have a baby and isn't sure how her body will respond, her first childbirth is likely to be the scariest to contemplate. Many women select the medicated, monitored route for first childbirth, then graduate to Lamaze for a second delivery. If they have already had a successful Lamaze birth, or live in an area like California where Bradley is very popular, they may be ready to look into Bradley for a second childbirth—

perhaps even a first! For those with enough self-confidence, it may be the most rewarding natural childbirth method available in the United States.

To register for classes: Write to Bradley Method, P. O. Box 5224, Sherman Oaks, California 91413, or call 213–788-6662.

A PERSONAL GROWTH EXPERIENCE

As early as 1945, Dr. Helene Deutsch, an eminent psychoanalyst, questioned the way anesthesia was robbing women of the opportunity for self-development through childbirth. She believed that during childbirth a kind of altered state of consciousness occurs that makes unconscious material more accessible to the conscious mind, and that during childbirth the mother reaffirms her psychic connections with her own mother and mothering. She felt that actively mastering the labor experience can be both cathartic and ego-strengthening.

Contemporary childbirth educators who emphasize the psychotherapeutic effects of childbirth believe that a good childbirth experience can help women free themselves from sexual inhibitions that create marital tension during pregnancy and fear of childbirth itself. Sheila Kitzinger in England and Lester Hazell in California both candidly discuss such taboo areas as mutual masturbation, mutual sexual massage, and the physical pleasures of childbirth and breast-feeding in their classes and books (see Bibliography). In Kitzinger's childbirth philosophy called the "psycho-sexual approach:" "Pregnancy is, or can be, an occasion for spectacular emotional growth, involving as it often does a series of crises as the expectant mother gradually comes to terms with her new identity. . . . It's a second adolescence. Far from confining itself to teaching a set of physiological tricks, preparation for childbirth can teach a woman how to trust herself."

In her books, Kitzinger teaches women to "swim" over the wave of a contraction and not be enveloped by it. She has discovered an association between the vaginal and mouth muscles: "When a woman proves tense in the region of the pelvic floor, she can often be helped to relax by teaching her to relax her mouth and jaw." She recommends relaxed smiling with lips parted, as the head is crowning and the baby is being born.

Lester Hazell, a practicing transactional analyst as well as a natural-childbirth teacher, also emphasizes the emotional aspects of the child-birth experience: "Childbirth is a transcendental experience . . . often compared to a sexual orgasm. It is a characteristic of labor, like sexual intercourse, to require the best a woman has to give if she is to get the most out of it. In any event, labor strips her of her veneer. It is a nitty-gritty experience in which a woman encounters herself at her core."

She also recommends dealing realistically with the limitations of in-tercourse in preganancy. "Undesired intercourse can cause morning sickness," she points out. "Massage can communicate feelings. . . . Mutual acceptance and enjoyment of one another's masturbation is an important part of a couple's sexual adjustment. . . . We are sexual beings from birth to death. . . . Both sexes are capable of experiencing a far wider ability to be sexual. Pregnancy offers the chance to grow, to dis-solve old barriers, and to become more authentic people."

This open exploration of sexual feelings and physical sensations is a great advance in childbirth education. Many women are ashamed to dis-cuss sexual matters with male obstetricians, and for some, the inhibition is much deeper—they cannot even discuss sex openly with their mates. Rather than causing loneliness, fear, and depression, the physical changes of pregnancy can lead to greater marital and sexual communica-tion and intimacy, and increase the woman's feelings of strength and pleasure in her body. Self-understanding and self-acceptance in every area increases psychological health and emotional resilience.

Because of her interest in psychological growth, Hazell goes beyond the sexual area to help women achieve self-knowledge. She suggests learning, in advance, how you're likely to behave when you're about to deliver the baby:

"We all use our automatic pilot under stress," she points out. "One way is to 'be nice,' another is to 'be perfect.' A third is to 'hurry up,' and a fourth to 'be strong.' The fifth is to 'try hard.' " Using her formulation, take a moment to think about your own response to stress situations. Do you always try to be nice? Or are you the strong, silent, martyr type? Do you worry constantly that you won't do the job well and fear failures? By knowing yourself better, you can control these automatic responses that are used to impress others; you can relax instead and act the way you really feel. And that's the best way to have a fulfilling childbirth ex-perience!

What delights me most about the philosophy of Kitzinger and Hazell is that it views the pregnant woman as a whole individual rather than as a patient or a wife. The more "person-centeredness" is developed in pregnancy, the more expressive a woman is likely to be from that point on. Her experiences as wife, childbearer, sexual being, and nursing mother will be enriched and more fruitful.

The best childbirth teachers of every persuasion are beginning to think along these lines. My suggestion is that you find a teacher who will relate to you as a growing, changing, and autonomous individual who is experiencing one of the biggest adventures in her life.

DOCTOR-CENTERED NATURAL CHILDBIRTH

Many women are not ready for the "full growth experience." What they want is the guidance of a strong, fatherly doctor they can rely on and trust. We have all grown up with this tradition, and if you feel you still need that kind of relationship in natural childbirth, find a doctor who is a warm humanist who inspires enough trust and confidence to allay the "parturiphobia" (fear of childbirth) that plagues many of us.

Dr. Daniel Friedman of Lawrence, New York, is an example of that kind of doctor. He gets to know all his patients, sees them more frequently than most doctors do, and teaches his own childbirth preparation classes. His approach is "desensitization, group ventilation, and reality testing" during monthly meetings of all his patients. That means he prepares them for every possible problem that might come up and encourages open discussion and questions. After delivery, he invites some of the couples back to share their experiences with a new group, and he doesn't necessarily select those who had the most uneventful and problem-free experiences!

Friedman refers couples to every possible enrichment that the community offers: prepartum courses, postpartum supports, sensitivity training, La Leche League. (Some of these will be described in Part IV.) He is open to new ideas, involved in his own research, and encourages and supports the innovative work of others.

Four important stress points of modern hospital delivery are highlighted in his course. First, *false labor*—"When is it time to go to the hospital?" Second, *reactions to the hospitalization*—"Many women's contractions magically stop when they're about to be admitted." Third *transition stage*—"When the baby's head starts to descend through the incompletely dilated cervix, 7–9 centimeters, there may be discomfort which leads to tension, spasm of the pelvic musculature, and increased pain." He advises his patients to follow their own inclination to bear down, which automatically relaxes the pelvic musculature. During the last month of pregnancy and during early labor, Dr. Friedman repetitiously teaches the patient the proper expulsive techniques during vaginal examinations. Fourth, *expulsive stage*—"When the mother moves from the labor to the delivery room. This last stress point could be avoided entirely if hospitals improved their maternity units, and arranged for labor, delivery, and recovery to take place in the same room." A few hospitals now have this birthing room as part of their family-centered maternity care.

Dr. Friedman stays with the mother throughout labor and delivery and puts the baby in her arms right after birth, even before cutting the umbilical cord. The process is as supportive and emotionally fulfilling for the mother as possible.

Husbands are in the delivery room, and patients are kept informed of their progress, but, more than with other natural childbirths, this is the doctor's show. Everyone must accept his obstetrical practices. Friedman uses electronic fetal monitors routinely, for example. Since the hospital he delivers in has no rooming-in for the first twenty-four hours, mother and baby must be separated, except for feeding.

One of Dr. Friedman's patients told me, "I can hardly wait to have the next baby." "Still," she warned, "Dr. Friedman is not the best choice for a person who needs a lot of sympathy and handholding."

If you do choose doctor-centered childbirth, your comfort and confidence in the relationship are even more important than in the other methods. If you're the kind of person who is most comfortable with a strong authority figure (and many people are), find yourself a dedicated, intelligent, psychologically-oriented doctor you can respect, and *lean*.

THE RED CROSS PREPARATION

The Red Cross course, available in every community and known all over the world for more than fifty years, is very up to date and not to be overlooked. It is free except for materials. There are seven sessions, and all classes are taught by specially trained registered nurses.

Red Cross emphasizes safety, planning, nutrition and practice in such activities as buying a layette and baby supplies, and holding, bathing, feeding, and diapering the baby. Labor is discussed in detail and also the characteristics of a new baby. A Lamaze film is shown, since many of the participants also take a Lamaze preparation course at the same time. Helen Miles, director of Parenthood Programs for the Nassau County Red Cross, reports that "every bit of practical information is soaked up avidly. People leave feeling secure and well prepared."

Information about such things as taking the baby's temperature, interpreting cries, spotting illnesses, safety in the car, mouth-to-mouth resuscitation, and breast- and bottle-feeding is taught in hospitals after delivery, but it's a lot easier to absorb before the birth, when you have the time and are relaxed.

Learning to bathe the baby is part of the tradition of the Red Cross preparation classes. (Borgne Keith/Nassau Chapter of the American Red Cross)

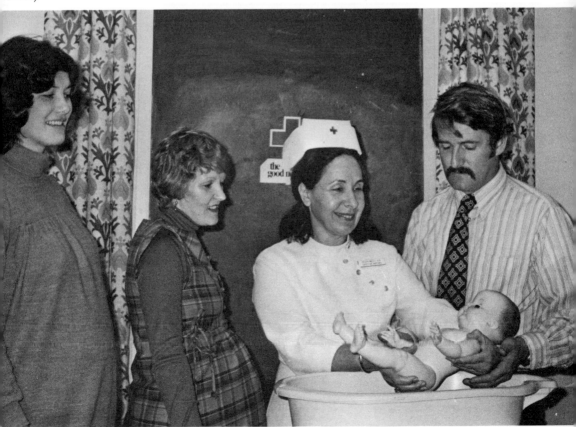

The last session of Mrs. Miles's course is devoted to "rearing a child of goodwill." It aims to increase awareness of the importance of transmitting tolerant racial and religious attitudes and is jointly sponsored by an interfaith organization in the community. There is an opportunity to continue postpartum with the same group to discuss handling everyday problems.

Call your local Red Cross chapter and ask what is included in the course in your own neighborhood. Is Lamaze preparation part of it? Is there a fee involved?

YOGIC CHILDBIRTH

Yoga is not a religion or one practice, but a set of disciplines (differing according to the type of yoga) with the same spiritual philosophy. The teaching covers every aspect of daily living. The aspects of childbirth and family life include methods of natural birth control and conscious conception; food preparation and eating practices; sexual, marital, and child-rearing practices; meditation and chanting. "We have a whole lifestyle to offer," says Sat Jivan Kaur Khalsa, a young mother and yoga instructor who, with her husband, leads a 3HO (Happy, Healthy, Holy Organization) Foundation ashram in Brooklyn, New York.

"Conscious conception" is an important part of spiritual childbirth. "Preparation-for-pregnancy workshops give people the opportunity to examine their motives and desires for having children as well as provide nutritional and herbal preparation for a healthy pregnancy," says Parvati of the Center for Family Growth in California.

All yogas are vegetarians and do not believe in as high a protein intake during pregnancy as other childbirth experts. Yet their nutritional counseling is aimed at helping mothers tune in to their own bodies and nutritional needs, and there is no requirement that participants be vegetarians. *Diet for a Small Planet,* a vegetarian cookbook, is on the recommended list for vegetarian students of the 3HO program, for example, and Adelle Davis's books are used to help the meat eaters.

Some yoga sects recommend sexual abstinence in the latter part of pregnancy and for the nine months to a year of breast-feeding. Others counsel complete sexual abstinence at all times except for purposes of conception, and still others believe in free sex play for a married couple.

However, yogic teachers do not try to impose these beliefs on outsiders. They individualize counseling to meet their students' needs.

Fees for counseling and classes are scaled low, and sometimes goods and services are bartered in exchange for the classes. This is important since there is a long series of classes that continue right through pregnancy. Women usually come in alone, but couples are not uncommon. Enrollment can be at any stage of pregnancy, the earlier the better. Arrangements differ according to the yoga center, but classes usually are in sets—of six, eight, or ten—which then are repeated at later stages of the pregnancy. "The prenatal yoga classes are on-going," says Parvati. "They can become a woman's daily ritual at home, and then classes provide new *pranayamas* [conscious breathing exercises], more and more advanced *asanas* [poses], and support for *sadhana* [spiritual practice] as the pregnancy progresses."

In some centers, women take outside Lamaze classes. This fits in with the yogic attitude—"Learn as much as possible and apply the techniques that work best for you."

The yoga approach to childbirth can be characterized as somewhere between Lamaze and Bradley, offering the spiritual perspective that helps a woman decide which one to use as the birth approaches. During delivery, she concentrates on being totally present, but also controls this awareness according to her tolerance and capacities. Thus, for example, she may choose to deflect her attention away from the contractions some times, and at others be fully involved in the experience. She uses meditation and chanting and the support of the whole group's spiritual participation, even though they may not be physically present in the birthing room.

According to Mrs. Khalsa, "A woman is master of her own fate. Her behavior causes its own effects. Within this perspective, a woman can handle childbirth in a serene and mature way."

Says Parvati, "It is the image and the expectations that a woman has about being a mother that tremendously affect her childbirth experience. Yogic childbirth education emphasizes the ability to create your own pain (and/or ecstasy) during the birthing experience."

A complete postpartum program is part of the yogic childbirth experience. It is recommended that women and their babies remain in seclusion for up to forty days, with a minimum of outside visitors. A *sevadar*, or helping person trained to join the woman and her husband in their home for this period of time, is part of the 3HO program. She prepares the necessary special foods and provides all the household help needed. A *sevadar* is characterized by Mrs. Khalsa as "a woman who learns to tune in and take care of someone selflessly." Most of these helpers are members of the 3HO ashrams, but outsiders also are trained to help their friends and family members after childbirth.

There is no exact way of counting the number of yogic childbirth classes available throughout the United States. They are becoming more numerous, however, and the 3HO group already has one hundred ashrams throughout the country, many offering childbirth instruction. Their members also teach at nearby community colleges. Other centers independent of 3HO, also are starting up, like the Center for Family Growth.

The broad curriculum of the Center for Family Growth indicates how rich the yogic childbirth education is. Among the classes and service offered in their countrylike setting are: conscious conception and natural birth control; prenatal yoga; massage for pregnancy; marriage, family, and child counseling (individual, couples, and groups); family herbal care; and new parents' workshops.

Other courses in the center are open to the entire community. These include various kinds of psychotherapy groups, homeopathy (a natural form of healing), herbs and nutrition, astrology (used for fertility counseling and for calculating the ideal time for couples to conceive their children). Since home birth is the expected choice, all yogic childbirth centers have individual and group classes to prepare properly for childbirth at home. The Center for Family Growth also offers a basic midwifery course. Instructors include an obstetrician well experienced in home births, a midwife who is a registered nurse, and a widely known lay midwife in California.

There may be other such centers. The Center for Family Growth group is interested in helping more get started and also will advise you where to find a resource close to your home. Some of these centers incorporate the yoga philosophy, while others embrace the psychotherapeutic and naturopathic aspects without the spiritual philosophy. The ICEA representative in your area (see Appendix I) also should be able to steer you to a "holistic center," if one exists in your community.

Obviously, yogic childbirth is a special experience not suitable for many women. Its recommendation that a woman follow her appetite rather than any nutritional guidelines requires a sensitivity to one's body

ieeds that may be obtained better in theory than in practical life. After
eating regular foods all her life, a young woman interested in yoga may
ake up vegetarian practices with great enthusiasm and overdo, just as
ther people try fasting, rice diets, or other extreme methods to attain
pirituality at the cost of their health. Unless a woman has found she can
emain healthy on the recommended yoga diet with its lower protein
intake for a considerable amount of time before pregnancy, I feel she
hould follow the protein recommendations outlined in chapter 2.

If you live in an ashram or communal home with the practical postpartum supports necessary for both mother and child, home birth can
vork out very well. Through the yoga teacher, you will be able to find a
qualified birth assistant, usually an experienced nurse-midwife, who will
come to your home. However, if you're planning a home birth on your
own, as a couple, it is *very important* to follow the recommendations in
chapter 11.

If you're the kind of person who is interested in meditation, in following the sexual- and life-styles of the yogas, then "spiritual" childbirth
nay help you have your baby with peace of mind. Only you know if you
need this kind of framework and whether pregnancy is the right time for
vou to find it.

Read: Prenatal Yoga and Natural Birth by Jeannine O'Brien Medvin
Parvati), Freestone Publishing Collective, 555 Highland Avenue, Penngrove, California 94951. This well-written explanation of yogic childbirth
s full of personal experiences and beautiful demonstration photographs
of preparatory exercises.

For further information and referral to a class, write to 3HO Founda-
ion, International (Kundalini yoga preparation), House of Guru Ram
Das, 1620 Preuss Road, Los Angeles, California 90035; tel: 213–550–9043.
Or Parvati, Center for Family Growth (synthesis of yogas), 555 High-
and Avenue, Penngrove, California 94951; tel: 707–795–5155.

FOLLOW YOUR FEELINGS

By now you're aware that there is no one "natural way." Natural childbirth does require mental and physical preparation, but this can be done
nformally at home as well as in a class. No one course of instruction is
best for everyone. Knowing about all of them means you can select the
one that seems to fit your own personality best.

You may be a Bradley type, with a profound dislike of being told by anyone what to do; you may feel strongly that childbirth belongs to you and your husband and that you want no interference by any medical authority. You may feel fairly confident of your ability to handle the normal stresses of childbirth and desire to experience it fully. You may also agree with Kitzinger and Hazell that natural childbirth is a personal growth experience. Their philosophy fits well within the Bradley framework.

Or you may be a Lamaze type who feels most supported in the egalitarian, optimistic atmosphere of the team approach. You want to be consulted about what is happening and being planned for you, but feel most comfortable about leaving medical decisions in the experts' hands. Of course, you want your chosen companion close to you throughout. You like the idea of deflecting attention away from contractions through

Keeping in tune with each other can make even a long labor easier.
(Mariette Pathy Allen)

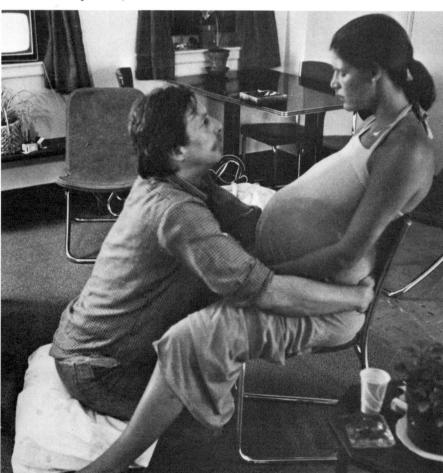

breathing and eye-focusing exercises, if it means getting through childbirth with dignity, control, and self-respect.

You may be a Dick-Read woman, wanting to know what to expect, desiring sympathetic and competent people to help you so you can get through without following any formalized system of breathing. You are choosing natural childbirth more for the baby's sake than for any ecstatic experience of your own. As long as your companion can be there, you will be comfortable in a hospital with a doctor you can trust.

If you believe you need the positive support of a trusted doctor more than exercises, breathing, and philosophy, then your ICEA representative will refer you to local natural-childbirth doctors, and the national offices of Bradley, Lamaze, and Dick-Read will add to that list. It will be up to you then to meet with several until you form the right "fit" in the relationship. In my opinion, a solid doctor-patient relationship, based on easy, candid communication, is a vital part of *any* successful childbirth.

If you find yourself attracted to the special spiritual experience of a yoga childbirth, by all means follow your impulse and discuss the method with a yoga childbirth teacher.

Each of these approaches is the right one for some people. Which is right for you? Read about them, talk about them, interview a number of teachers. Then, when your feelings jell, follow them.

The best kind of preparation is the one that offers just the right balance of reality and inspiration—that tells the whole, unvarnished truth about the stresses, discomforts, and emergencies that may arise in natural childbirth, particularly with twins or breech birth.

More women today are selecting midwives rather than obstetricians for natural childbirth. Most midwives are knowledgeable about all methods of natural childbirth and flexible about using whichever one you prefer. They will work out a delivery procedure—dimming lights, baby bath, etc.—that suits the couple. Also, the midwife will tell you where to find the natural-childbirth class that seems to suit your needs best, or will teach you herself. If you have contacted a nurse-midwife unit of a hospital or a privately practicing nurse-midwife before choosing your method of natural childbirth, use her as a good referral source to a teacher.

Most obstetricians are familiar only with the Lamaze method. Get in touch with the national organizations of the other methods for referrals to their classes. They also have lists of doctors who are familiar with and practice their method.

8

Breast, Bottle, or Both?

As a psychotherapist, I'm enthusiastic about breast-feeding. As a mother, I also am sensitive to the special problems breast-feeders have in today's world. In this chapter, I'll be discussing both, to help you decide for yourself whether breast-feeding is right, and possible, for you.

Only 25 percent of American babies are being breast-fed. It is just as important for bottle-feeders as breast-feeders to know how to feed their babies sensitively and how to tune in to their needs. Bottle-feeders have the same problems of loneliness, tiredness, and worry about whether they're reading the baby's body language correctly as their breast-feeding sisters. Both breast- and bottle-feeders need to learn how to obtain the fullest possible participation and cooperation of their husbands.

As both mother and psychotherapist, I have found that the difference between a happy and unhappy feeding relationship with your baby depends more on the outside supports you can arrange than on almost any other factor! Therefore, a good many of my suggestions show how to make the best possible use of your environment to help you succeed with whichever method you choose.

THE STORY OF INFANT FEEDING

Throughout history, the choice of feeding method and the style of feeding have depended on fashion and finances. In rich societies, such as ancient Rome, upper-class women often rejected breast-feeding on the advice of their doctors. Lower-class nursing mothers, called "wet nurses," were hired to do the job for them. These women often had to leave their own infants to be breast-fed by some compassionate neighbor or to survive on a "pap" food, like banana. In these class-stratified societies, some lucky babies were fed on demand in a leisurely and permissive manner whenever they seemed hungry. However, all in all, many more babies died of malnutrition.

In poor societies, most women had to work outside the home, so breast-feeding was very hard to manage. Infants were fed at the convenience of adults, and feeding times were cursory and brief. Often milk was eliminated from the diet altogether and babies were fed on pap food. Not surprisingly, more infants died in impoverished societies than in more affluent ones where mothers could stay home and breast-feed them.

About sixty years ago, both breast-feeding and demand feeding went into sharp decline in the United States—a decline that is slowly spreading to the rest of the world. Modern technology developed a cow's-milk formula that provided nourishment when breast milk was not available, and most infants thrived on it. Separating mothers and babies right after birth became the mode in hospitals, and sterilization made formula preparation safer and easier. It was a time when women went to work in stores and factories in large numbers. The media advertised and popularized bottle-feeding. Breast-feeders soon felt old-fashioned while bottle-feeding became so popular that the art of breast-feeding was almost lost in the United States.

Most of the world's babies continued to be breast-fed, however, and both breast-feeding and feeding on demand rather than by strict schedule are becoming fashionable again. About 25 percent of American women try breast-feeding now (up to 45 percent on the West Coast). However, we still have by far the lowest proportion of breast- to bottle-feeders in the entire world, and American women have considerable problems with breast-feeding. Many Americans have never seen a baby breast-fed since there remains a strong taboo against nursing in public. The "American" style of feeding remains the bottle, with a shift toward demand feeding and away from strict schedules.

Although about 90 percent of the world's women breast-feed, the length of nursing time is declining. In some cultures, babies are breast-fed for more than two years, but in increasing numbers of societies, solid feeding begins early and nursing is for less than a year. About ten years ago, some of the newly developing countries tried to copy our "modern way" of infant feeding—with disastrous results. Because of improper storage, sterilization and over-dilution, bottle-fed babies became sick and died. The United Nations, through its World Health Organization, began promoting breast-feeding with educational programs. In countries where governments actively educate for and support breast-feeding, it is successfully practiced by more than 95 percent of mothers.

Whether or not a woman breast-feeds in America depends on whether her friends do, her familiarity with breast-feeding, what she knows about its advantages and disadvantages, what her husband wants her to do, and what the doctor advises. The doctor's opinion, it has been found, depends more on how his wife fed their children than on any other factor. Doctors are like the rest of us—they grew up unfamiliar with breast-feeding. In medical school, they learn more about the management of a bottle baby than how to teach the techniques of breast-feeding.

Today an American mother no longer feels as deviant as her own mother might have if she breast-feeds, but she is likely to have more problems nursing successfully than her European, Asian, South American, or African sisters. Because we have small families and move about so frequently, young, inexperienced mothers find themselves isolated with their infants and left to learn infant feeding by trial and error. The United States is reported to have a less adequate "support system" for new mothers than any country in the world. Family isn't available to help, and even our hospital nurses and pediatricians often know too little about breast-feeding techniques to be of much assistance.

"I know what I want to do," a mother-to-be told me. "But I don't know how to do it. My girlfriend was breast-feeding, and the nurses just handed her the baby and walked away. When she asked what to do, one nurse said, 'Why don't you just give the baby a bottle?' That's what I'm afraid will happen to me."

Another problem breast-feeders face is that until recently many doctors overemphasized weight gain and schedules for the new baby, and suggested weaning as soon as the mother complained or asked for help. That's because pediatricians knew more about handling babies' upsets from formulas than about overcoming breast-feeding problems.

Despite an unsupportive environment, many more women today are turning to the "natural way." Media information about nursing is increasing, largely due to the efforts of La Leche League, the breast-feeding self-help organization that reaches more than a million women a year with help, advice, encouragement, and information. Some doctors actively support nursing mothers by hiring nurses who are experienced breast-feeders to advise their patients or else refer them to the local La Leche League chapter. Slowly the art of breast-feeding is being revived.

Many women still are afraid to try breast-feeding. They too easily accept the ignorant opinion that there are no special advantages to breast-feeding and that they are probably too "high strung" to nurse successfully. Why 97 percent of Israeli women are not too high strung, why Swedish and Japanese women seem to have just the right temperament for it, are questions never raised in these discussions. Without familiarity, environmental support, and medical encouragement, the feeding method that used to be the most natural and easy in the world now seems as formidable as climbing a mountain.

BOTTLE-FEEDING:
ADVANTAGES AND DISADVANTAGES

In comparison to breast-feeding, bottle-feeding is promoted as being problem-free. Most babies do thrive on formulas, and infant survival no longer depends on mothers who are able or willing to breast-feed. It is socially permissible to bottle-feed a baby on a train, at the beach, in the park, but it's not easy to breast-feed publicly. There's no doubt that a nursing mother feels more constrained and less mobile than her bottle-feeding sister. But ingenuity makes public nursing possible, and the taboo against it is slowly disappearing as breast-feeding becomes more familiar and commonplace.

One concern about breast-feeding is that the mother carries the total responsibility for the survival of her baby. What if she becomes ill or is called away? There are answers. Breast-feeding babies can adjust to bottles temporarily and, if the mother is friendly with the La Leche women in her neighborhood, chances are that another woman will breast-feed the baby for her in an emergency.

At worst, your bottle-fed baby will have some trouble digesting a particular formula. Even if he's allergic to all cow's-milk formulas, soybean substitutes have been developed that will nourish him adequately. Some babies even seem to thrive on cow's milk, taken straight from the refrigerator, from birth on. However, you can't know before your baby comes whether his digestion will tolerate these substitutes. Babies develop a wide variety of disorders—general crankiness, gassiness, and even complete intolerance—on cow's milk.

Many people bottle-feed because they've heard that bottle babies sleep longer between feedings. Some do, some don't. When it's true, it's because cow's milk takes longer to digest than human milk. But the best schedule breaks down as soon as digestive problems arise, and with bottle-feeders they are not uncommon.

Your choice of feeding method and style of feeding will *not* determine how quickly the baby moves into a day-night schedule that is convenient to grown-ups. No matter what you do, you may end up saying, as one woman did, "My first two babies were dolls, but this one is impossible. He sleeps all day and wants to play all night." The baby's digestive system, his temperament, the peacefulness of the room in which he sleeps, all help determine how successful nighttime sleep scheduling will be. Some babies—both breast- *and* bottle-fed—sleep all night within weeks of birth. (Unless the baby isn't gaining weight properly, that's one feeding you'll never wake him up for!) Others resist giving up a night feeding for months, and also tend to wake with teething pain well into the second year. Keep in mind that being anxious, hovering over the baby, and picking him up for feeding every time he makes a sound won't help him adjust to a good schedule on his own. Many healthy babies will fall back to sleep in a minute or two if they are mature enough physically not to need a feeding.

One difficulty with bottle-feeding that frequently is glossed over is finding the magic nipple hole size that gives the baby sufficient sucking exercise and is not so small that he becomes frustrated and exhausted during feeding. You have to enlarge the nipple hole by trial and error as the baby grows, increasing the flow just enough so he won't gag or vomit excess milk too often.

Bottle-fed babies generally get more gas pains than those who are breast-fed since they suck in air with their milk. Some of the new nipples attempt to deal with this problem through improved design. Some bottle-fed babies also get eczema, which is an itchy skin disorder, or other symptoms of allergy to cow's milk. As long as the baby can tolerate minor symptoms, most doctors will not experiment with changing formulas, so it's up to the mother to comfort the fretful child. When celiac disease, a serious digestive problem due to slow development of the digestive system, is known to be in the family history on either the mother's or the father's side, doctors recommend breast-feeding to avoid it.

The greatest advantage to bottle-feeding is that you know the baby is full. That is no small thing to us Americans. Our babies grow so fat, even in the first year of life, that they need to be put on skim-milk diets. Mothers with plenty of breast milk are not concerned about this problem, but for those with scanty supplies and fussy babies it can be an escalating concern. More than one woman has become anxious enough about it to seek psychological help. One patient told me, "I dream that the baby talks to me. She says, 'Stupid, why don't you give me a bottle?' " Unfortunately, when the mother weaned her baby to a bottle, the nightmares didn't go away. Instead she dreamed the baby said, "Stupid, why don't you punch a hole in the nipple?" The problem is as much in the mother's perception as in the baby's response. However, by and large, formula-fed babies *are* more placid and content, less demanding of constant attention.

And they grow! Recent generations of Americans, mostly bottle-fed, are much taller and bigger-boned than their parents. Much of this difference is due to improved nutrition throughout childhood, but some seems to be the result of drinking so much cow's milk. Bottle-fed babies are known to grow more rapidly and gain more weight in infancy than most breast-fed babies.

BREAST-FEEDING:
ADVANTAGES AND DISADVANTAGES

The reason breast-fed babies eat so frequently in the first weeks and months is that they get full quickly, digest rapidly, and are ready for the next feeding in less than two hours. Even babies whose mothers have bountiful supplies of milk nurse frequently, except for one or two longer sleep periods during the day that (the mothers hope) will combine eventually to give them a night's sleep.

Some women find it harder to interpret the needs of breast-fed babies. They are awake more than bottle babies and get used to playing and communicating. They're not so digestion-centered. Are they hungry or just asking for holding and cuddling? These babies seem to thrive on attention as much as on food. It is delightful to watch them with their mothers—demanding eye contact, verbalizing in a surprisingly mature way. It is a mistake to compare their developmental pattern to that of the placid, doll-like, sleepy bottle-fed baby.

Even within each feeding method infants develop very differently, so it is clear that the method of feeding is only part of the reason for a baby's behavior. Compare breast-fed babies, for example. Some are eager to nurse and get right down to business. Others are more playful. Some fall asleep in the middle of a feeding—it seems to take forever for them to finish. These differences are both genetic and environmental (depending on the baby's experience in the womb and during birth).

Every baby is an individual from birth, entitled to his or her own personality. Feeding problems begin when mothers prod babies to change their ways. Think about your own personality and your husband's. You know how set in your ways you are, with your own characteristics. So is a baby. The feeding relationship works out best when you can accept your baby as he is. After all, the baby also has to learn to adjust to you. He holds you and caresses your skin during feedings, responds when you put a nipple in his mouth. Infant feeding is a two-way adjustment, a give-and-take between two distinct personalities.

A most important advantage of breast-feeding is the quality of the sucking experience. Prolonged sucking develops relaxed breathing, good muscular coordination, proper facial development, and the correct alignment of dental arches and palates. Sucking needs of both breast and bottle babies can be supplemented by using pacifiers, which help the baby relax without having to stuff his stomach. But breast sucking is most satisfying for the baby because he can regulate the amount of intake exactly. He can suck in a little milk without overeating and vomiting, as a strong-sucking bottle baby might do. The sucking exercise in infancy has been found to lead to decreased respiratory illness later in life, and psychologists find that breast-fed babies are more secure.

There are documented advantages for the mother, too, both physical and psychological. The uterus returns to normal size more quickly for breast-feeders, and there is less postpartum bleeding. Although there is no definitive answer about whether the incidence of breast cancer is lower in breast-feeders than in bottle-feeders, studies do indicate there may be a connection. Societies in which babies are routinely nursed have a lower rate of breast cancer. Not just lactation, but prolonged breast-feeding, seems to be related to prevention of breast cancer.

There is also a positive relationship between breast-feeding and the reestablishment of a good marital relationship after the baby's birth. Breast-feeders are less "touchy" about physical contact, despite any discomfort of heavy or leaky breasts, because they have intimate skin con-

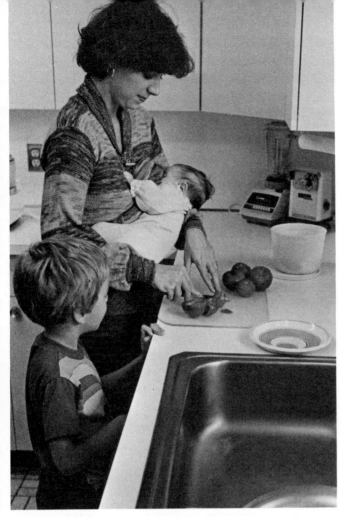

Breast-feeding can easily become a part of regular home activities. (Alison Ehrlich Wachstein, from Pregnant Moments, *Morgan & Morgan, 1978)*

tact with the baby right after birth. Many resume sexual relations more quickly and easily than bottle-feeders. Since *complete* breast-feeding usually stops ovulation, nursing a baby often is advocated as a natural method of spacing babies.

FACTS ABOUT BREAST MILK

There are some outstanding advantages of breast milk over formula. In the first few days of nursing, a yellowish liquid called colostrum is secreted in the breast. This valuable liquid provides the baby with his mother's current immunities to infection. He also is much less likely to catch viruses and infections circulating in the neighborhood since his mother's breast milk continues to supply antibodies to fight new sources of infection in the environment.

Since breast milk is 100 percent digestible, diarrhea, constipation, and eczema are much less likely and less severe if they do occur. Allergies need not be a concern, unless foods are being used as a supplement.

Unfortunately, many American babies begin eating solids at two weeks of age, which is much too early to be safe. Before the baby's digestive system is mature, any food can upset it, or create allergies later in life. Allergists are reporting banana allergies in teenagers, for example, and banana has traditionally been used as the safest, most easily digestible food in early infant feeding.

One condition of allergic response to a mother's milk was recently discovered by neonatologist Lawrence Gartner of Albert Einstein College of Medicine in New York. A component of the mother's milk inhibits the natural function of an enzyme in the baby's liver, and jaundice results. The condition is rarely dangerous and often is passed over without being noticed, since mothers rarely recognize jaundice (the baby just looks rosier than usual). Dr. Gartner advises that if this condition occurs, the mother should stop breast-feeding for a few days, until her doctor is sure that the toxic level has dropped. Then she should resume breast-feeding. There are too many advantages—immunological and nutritional—to give up breast feeding.

There is no known allergy to breast milk, although up to 10 percent of babies are allergic to cow's milk and some are even allergic to soybean formula. A very few babies cannot digest any milk at all, but their condition is discoverable at birth in routine tests.

When a mother is very tense, her baby may refuse to nurse, cry, and make faces as if the taste of the milk is bothering him. When the tension is dispelled, the milk is perfectly good, whether it looks creamy or watery. The color and consistency depend on the fat content, but all mother's milk is good for the baby, and his own mother's milk provides the best protection against infection. At the start of nursing, the milk often appears more watery, while the "hindmilk," at the end, is richest in caloric content.

Many women today are concerned about transmitting environmental pollutants to the baby through their breast milk. This is happening, since pollutants collect in human fat and are transmitted in breast milk. It is important to avoid additives, hairsprays, and all other known environmental pollutants while you are breast-feeding. However, after studying pollutants in breast milk, the Senate Subcommittee on Health and Scientific Research said in June 1977, "There is no reason at this time to discontinue breast-feeding." Experts like Dr. Gartner are convinced that the outstanding immunological, nutritional, emotional, and psychological advantages of breast-feeding far outweigh the disadvantage of pollution.

If you're concerned about pollutants and plan to breast-feed, follow these La Leche League recommendations:

1. Avoid using insecticides.
2. Avoid animal fat as much as possible, and cut the fat from your meat.
3. Wash fruits and vegetables thoroughly before eating.
4. Avoid fish from waters known to be contaminated.

La Leche League will send you the latest findings on *Contaminants in Human Milk* if you will write to them in Franklin Park, Illinois, and ask for Leaflet 78A. (Send a self-addressed, stamped envelope).

You can do a great deal to decrease pollutants in your breast milk by avoiding processed foods with chemical additives and limiting your intake of nicotine, caffeine, and alcohol.

EMOTIONAL STRESSES OF INFANT FEEDING

If a baby is born with a good digestion and easygoing temperament, if the mother is relaxed and secure, infant feeding will go easily. Often it does. Sometimes, however, there is considerable stress in the feeding relationship in the early months. Part of the reason is our own expectations. We were raised to believe that there is an answer to every problem, if only we are smart enough and efficient enough to find it. In interpersonal situations, however, problems very often need time to work themselves out. Unfortunately, we get this perspective only through experience and maturity, after spending months floundering about trying to find the perfect answer.

In the first weeks and months, babies have growth spurts every few weeks. After being perfectly content on the breast or bottle, suddenly they begin to cry miserably, as if they were starving to death. If you're expecting these growth spurts, you can handle them with aplomb. Breast-feeders can nurse more frequently or add a bit of formula as a supplement to nursing—or both—and things will soon settle down again. Bottle-feeders can forget about their schedules for a few days and feed the baby on demand.

If you're taken by surprise, however, growth spurts can create mountainous problems. The breast-feeder will be tempted to go to the closest drugstore, stock up on formula, hand the baby to her husband, forget about the nursing, and go to sleep. Bottle-feeders will call their pediatricians in a panic and begin solid feeding, or change to another formula on his advice.

The baby will probably be content—for a while. Then, on the bottle or new formula, he will scream again. Maybe he is having a new growth spurt, maybe the new food is troubling his digestion. No matter what the advertisements say or the doctor tells you, it is your baby's temperament, digestive system, and developmental needs that determine his response to feeding. Figuring out what the baby wants and needs at any particular time is harder than most people expect.

Some mothers express regret after they wean the baby on an impulse. It isn't impossible to change your mind and unwean, but it does take a great deal of determination to urge the breast on a baby after he's had the experience of a full belly with practically no exertion. It's worth

Some activities, like graduate level courses, may be too hard to balance easily with new motherhood. (Alison Ehrlich Wachstein, from Pregnant Moments, *Morgan & Morgan, 1978)*

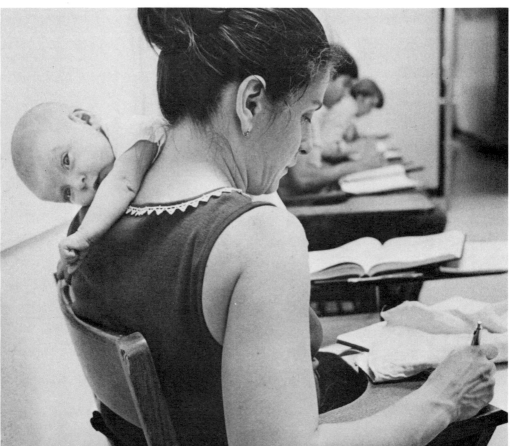

trying, however, and some babies do cooperate. Every baby is different, just as every mother's motivation is different. Some babies are stubborn from the minute they're born. Others are remarkably malleable and a persistent mother can accomplish almost anything.

A NEW LIFE-STYLE

The slow, responsibility-laden pace of life is probably the hardest thing to adjust to as a new mother. Feeding and tending the baby is a round-the-clock activity for the first months. It is wise to plan for fulfilling, relaxing at-home activities such as reading, painting, sewing, or decorating the apartment. Otherwise you're likely to get restless, bored, even jumpy and claustrophobic—and escalating tension can destroy the pleasure and successful adjustment of the infant-feeding relationship.

What is experienced as an advantage by one mother in this new life-style is felt as a tremendous disadvantage by another. For example, an on-demand breast-feeder hardly will be able to leave home for her own recreation and socialization until the baby develops his own schedule. If she has many home-bound projects and friendly, compatible adult companionship whenever she wants some, this period will be particularly precious and happily spent. But if she is restlessly waiting for an opportunity to get out shopping, dancing, to the beauty parlor, to the museum, she will feel tied down and antagonistic toward the baby.

Sleeping through the night usually is impossible for a while. In retrospect, this period is brief, but for some women, it will be experienced as excruciating. The lucky women are those who can slip easily into a pattern of napping between feedings, while the baby sleeps.

Constant interaction and contact are wonderful for the baby, but some women find it impossible to relax unless they're completely alone. They feel lonesome when the baby is asleep and anxious for him to get up so they can have something to do. Then they hardly can wait for him to go off to sleep again. Adult companionship is a tremendous relief for these women—even for an hour or two. Baby-sitters, so the mother can get out, are also a necessity when the mother is becoming depressed and exhausted with anxiety and isolation.

A breast-feeder is less likely to be bored and lonesome than a bottle-feeder simply because she is kept busier. The constant feeding and interaction with the baby is exhausting, but it's a lot easier emotionally than hovering over a sleeping baby, waiting for him to get up.

Breast-feeders have the emotional advantage of feeling special and irreplaceable. When a feeding goes well, when the baby has a good day, there is a unique feeling of success and accomplishment. Whenever the baby cries, the breast-feeder serenely offers her breast—for feeding or for comfort—knowing she is right on target.

It is not uncommon for the breast-feeder to have considerable rebellious feelings about having to watch her diet, her rest, and her exercise, just as she did during pregnancy. Impulses to crash-diet, to eat junk foods, will obsess some breast-feeders in the early months. They may be tempted to wean the baby because their breasts are uncomfortably full or too large to fit well into their prepregnancy wardrobes. It helps to set a limited breast-feeding goal when you start so you won't feel stuck interminably. After about six weeks, you will be able to let down a little, go out between feedings, even skip a feeding by leaving your milk in a bottle or having your husband, friend, or relative give the baby some formula. When the time you have preset in your mind is up, you may very well decide to keep breast-feeding for another month or two.

I cannot emphasize too strongly that sensitive infant feeding, by a mother who cares for and responds to her baby and is trying to do the best job she can, is a difficult and tiring job. An intimate human relationship is being worked out. New skills are being learned. Try not to be perfectionistic and hard on yourself if things don't go smoothly. If you know that problems will arise, you won't feel like a failure when they do. Your goal is to keep functioning, and it's important to give yourself what you need to keep going. "If I have a baby-sitter, even for an hour or two, a couple of times a week, I'm all right," one mother told me. "I just go to the drugstore, eat a bagel, and drink some coffee and read a paper, like I used to do when I was working. I walk around, look into shop windows, and really breathe. After seeing the world, I come back home again and I can look at the baby."

ORAL ANXIETY

A common psychological problem is oral anxiety. New mothers sometimes are afraid the baby is starving when he cries. Some psychologists believe that the origin of this condition is in our own childhood experiences. Too many of us were fed on rigid schedules by inexperienced mothers who followed doctors' orders; they were told they would spoil us if we were fed on demand. Times and styles of feeding have changed, but sometimes scars remain.

When these women hear a baby—any baby—cry, they tend to get agitated. Once they are mothers, they worry inordinately about whether they are feeding the baby correctly, enough, or too much. Having wish-fulfillment dreams that the baby can communicate his needs is not uncommon. Others break down and cry with the baby and feel inadequate to carry the feeding responsibility alone. In extreme situations, they may wish the baby dead—even though, obviously, they are not the sorts of mothers who would ever hurt a baby. Women with oral anxiety take it out on themselves instead. They may lie awake all night, waiting for the baby to call, so that he will not cry with hunger pangs. As their children grow, if they don't overcome the problem, they overfeed, overprotect, and are oversolicitous of them.

For most women, the problem is over as soon as the baby is big enough to communicate in words. So, even if you think you may over-react to a baby's tears, consider it a mixed blessing. Orally anxious women often make the best, most responsive, and sensitive mothers once they overcome their terror of the feeding responsibility. They do tend to overfeed their babies, however, because they feel so secure and happy during feeding time. It's a good idea to find other outlets for mothering feelings with a young baby—such as playing with him and holding him—or he will surely get fat!

For the orally anxious mother, the concept of "modified demand"—letting the baby fuss, if not cry, and slowly stretching out the time between feedings—is intolerable. The mother should follow her feelings and pick up her baby whenever he needs attention. Soon she'll learn to distinguish between hunger and other needs. As the baby matures, the times between feedings will stretch by themselves. Her frequent contacts with the baby will relieve her anxiety, help her milk "let down" if she is breast-feeding, and make her feel more adequate as a mother.

Using a supplementary bottle when the baby cries *after* a breast-feeding can be relieving for the mother who worries that the baby may still be hungry. Often, he will take a little nip, burp once or twice, and fall asleep fully satisfied. Learning to feed a baby is a trial-and-error process, and checking in this fashion whether the baby is still hungry will relieve a mother's anxiety and often help her to continue breast-feeding.

COMBINING BREAST AND BOTTLE

Some breast-feeding experts frown on the practice of using either supplementary bottles (after a feeding) or complementary bottles (offered as a substitute for a breast-feeding). They fear that its usefulness will backfire, that once this practice starts, the breast-feeding will soon terminate.

In my opinion, success with combined feeding depends on the motivation of the mother who uses it. If, unconsciously, she's looking for a way to stop breast-feeding, she'll begin to substitute bottles for the breast more and more frequently. Since this is the best way to wean a baby (much better than stopping suddenly!), it certainly is not harmful. When the mother is using bottles for temporary relief, combined feeding will refresh her and enable her to continue breast-feeding. If she really wants to breast-feed, the only thing that will terminate is her anxiety and exhaustion, not the nursing.

Many American women are "partial lactators," that is, they combine breast, bottle, and solid feeding after the first months. This combination works well *if* the breast-feeding has been firmly established first and if the mother is eager to continue breast-feeding. Every situation is different and needs to be worked out to suit the nursing pair.

In America, total breast-feeding for nine months to a year is still rare, although it is common in many other societies and excellent for the baby. Don't push yourself to reach any rigid standard; it's far better to breast-feed within the limits of your own tolerance. Your first experience with the method may be briefer and more difficult than you expect, but as you gain mothering experience, breast-feeding will get easier and easier. The major problems, you will realize in retrospect, came from your anxiety rather than from insufficient milk. With this knowledge, the next time around, you will be able to breast-feed longer, using fewer supplements.

BREASTFEEDING AND MOTHERLINESS

A major concern of many women before the baby comes is that they will not be able to tolerate the constant intimacy with the baby, and that they will feel tied down at home and bored. After childbirth, particularly if it's been traumatic, some women do indeed have these feelings. In some, they even lead to postpartum depression.

However, many women who anticipate having these feelings don't ever get them. They find staying home with the baby a joy. It's being away from the baby they can't bear. They have a constant longing to get back, even on a rare evening out. Their genuine enjoyment of the interminable hours of baby care is surprising to an outsider, considering their previous life-styles and unfamiliarity with babies.

A major reason for this successful, rapid adaptation to the routines and responsibilities of motherhood is a psychological and biological phenomenon called *bonding*, which transforms ordinary adults into motherly and fatherly types.

From the baby's point of view, bonding means getting immediately attached to the mother, recognizing her, depending on her completely. In the fuzzy bliss of the early mother-child relationship, the mother is the magic person who always comes when baby cries, who always knows what he wants and gives it immediately. Since fathers are more actively involved with babies today, interacting in the same intimate, responsive way, some babies are fortunate enough to bond with both parents. They are twice blessed.

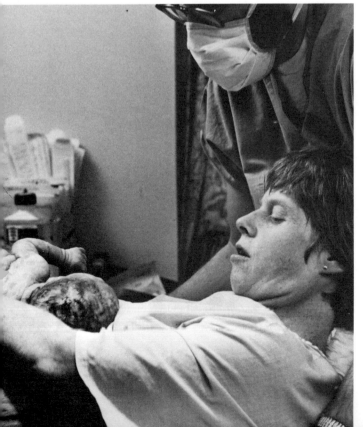

Immediately after drug-free childbirth mother and baby are intent on bonding. (From the Parenting Pictures film: The Bonding Birth Experience, *Courter Films and Associates)*

For a mother, bonding is like falling in love. The first euphoric hour after a drug-free childbirth, when the mother begins breast-feeding, is the perfect time for strong bonding. Other opportunities arise again and again for both breast- and bottle-feeders, particularly during feeding times. The mother feels as if her heart opens up. There is a rush of tender feeling for the baby, who seems perfection itself. Once this love is felt, the relationship is established, and the mother yearns to be with the baby whenever they're apart. She wants to hold him, thinks about him, and talks about him interminably. She even feels jealous when he smiles at someone else. She becomes sensitive to the baby's moods and communications, learns to "read" his cries and body language. Through bonding, the mother becomes motivated to develop that unique combination of responsive qualities we call "motherliness."

Breast-feeding sets the best conditions for strong bonding. One lactation hormone, prolactin, produces a vague craving for contact that is best soothed by mothering the baby. Another hormone, oxytocin, also is produced to "let down" the milk. This hormone, oxytocin, relaxes the woman and opens the ducts that make her milk available to the baby. Both hormones provide the physical stimuli for close contact. It's lucky they do, since mother and baby will be spending so much time together the first year. This constant emotional and physical contact is wonderful for the baby. If you feel you would like to have this constant intimacy with your baby, I recommend you try breast-feeding. Instead of being separated by the mechanics of bottle-feeding, you will find that your time together is much more meaningful and enjoyable.

A PERSONAL AFFAIR

Now is when you should make your choices, while there is plenty of time to consider the issues. Your best choice is the one based on a realistic balance of your own goals and personality and a baby's needs.

A lot of your motherliness will be expressed through feeding. Before you and the baby can communicate in other ways, your feelings will come through in your body language as you feed him. The quality of your relationship as well as the way he grows and develops will be affected by the feeding decisions you make now. They are likely to affect your life-style, your daily routine, and, ultimately, your feelings about being a mother.

Here are some questions to ask yourself now, before the baby comes. They are designed to help you think the issues through. Keep in mind that you do not have to come up with any final answers or definite commitments. "I don't know" means you're leaving yourself room to make up your mind later on, when you're with the baby. Your experience while giving birth, your state of mind afterward, the baby's experience getting born, and his innate personality are all factors that will ultimately influence your feeding relationship.

QUESTIONS TO ASK YOURSELF

Think about these questions and discuss them with the important people in your life. Even the experts differ on some of the answers, as you will see in the discussion following this questionnaire.

1. Would I rather feed the baby whenever he is hungry or do I want to aim for a schedule?

2. Do I want to limit the time of each feeding, particularly if I breast-feed, or let the baby set the pace completely?

3. If I am repelled by breast-feeding, do I want to try it for the baby's sake?

4. If I think, or have been told, that I am too high-strung, do I want to try breast-feeding anyway?

5. Do I want to begin breast-feeding if I know in advance that I will be stopping early? Will this upset the baby?

6. How will my husband react when I breast-feed? Will he be actively supportive, just put up with it, or hate it?

7. Will breast-feeding hinder my work, my sex life, my social life more or less than bottle-feeding?

8. Do I want to combine breast- and bottle-feeding? Why?

9. How do I feel about pacifiers for additional sucking for the baby?

10. How do I feel about weaning to a bottle? To a cup?

Answers to many of these questions differ, even among experts. Most agree that American babies get solid food far too early. They also say that constant response and attention to a baby in the first year will not spoil him. Schedules are not character-building, just convenient for adults. They will urge you to allow the baby plenty of sucking, for exercise and emotional satisfaction.

Breast-feeding experts point out the logical fact that the more you nurse, the more milk you produce. The more you skip feedings, the less likely you are to have enough to satisfy a growing baby. However, they also will tell you that times will arise (for example, during the growth spurts previously mentioned) when you will not have enough milk to satisfy the baby unless you nurse almost constantly for twenty-four hours. Some women use supplementary bottles to help them through these trying days. It is less important what you do than that you avoid panicking and precipitous weaning.

I hope all the experts you talk to and read will emphasize the uniqueness of each feeding relationship. It is a singular balance of both parties' needs. That is why it's called a *relationship*. You cannot blueprint the give-and-take between two people.

After a while, babies will be able to accept attention from other people, but at first their mother is their one and only love. And mothers can become depressed and exhausted if they respond to the baby at the cost of their own basic needs. If a woman gives up privacy, adult intimacy, sex, and fun, her relationship with the baby finally will suffer too.

INCREASED SELF-AWARENESS

Now think about your life-style, your goals as a mother, and, particularly, your personality. Perfection is impossible to achieve in infant feeding, so don't even try. Instead, discover yourself and candidly face your limitations. Answer the questions that follow as honestly as you can. Try to cue into your own feelings as sensitively right now as you will, later on, to the baby's.

1. How confident am I in my ability to be a good mother?
2. How much of my time and energy do I want to spend mothering?
3. What are my favorite recreations? How does a baby fit in?
4. For me, does a vacation mean being away from the baby?
5. For my husband, does a vacation mean being away from the baby? Do I want vacations?

6. How much do I care about having a fashionable figure and wardrobe and places to go where I can show them off?

7. Will I get bored at home?

8. How do I react when my sleep is interrupted? Can I nap?

9. Do I want help with the baby care? What kind of help? Will breast-feeding mean getting less help than I want?

10. For mothers of other children: What would I like to do differently this time in infant feeding?

Women's confidence before childbirth, particularly about whether they will be able to handle infant feeding, varies a great deal. It has been found that previous confidence has no relation to later success in infant feeding. In fact, if confidence means not learning about infant feeding in advance, not setting up the environmental conditions that might otherwise be possible, too much false confidence beforehand will result in plummeting disappointment later on.

If you're aware that you need more help and information, now is the time to get it. With every good book you read, every sound arrangement you make, your feelings of anxiety and apprehension will lessen.

Perhaps because of peer pressure, or the women's movement, some young women today are embarrassed to admit—to themselves, their husbands, their friends—that they want to be full-time mothers. For many years, it has been the woman who wanted to work outside the home, to continue her career while her children were small, who felt deviant. Times and fashions change, but women remain individuals. They are entitled to make their own choices and lead their lives in the ways that will be most fulfilling for themselves.

Of course, realistic limitations on free choice do shape mothering opportunities. Many women are obliged to return to work and contribute to family finances. Some women have no one to support them. They are unmarried and live on their own. No matter how much they might like to stay home, they have to arrange for someone else to take over infant care for them.

If you're fortunate enough to have free choice, exercise it. During pregnancy is the time to make your feelings known to the people who will be affected by your decision. Their cooperation and support will mean a great deal to you and strengthen your feelings for them. Communication is the key here.

Thinking about what you like to do in your free time might sound frivolous, but it's one of the best possible preparations for motherhood. The women who find early infant care easiest are those who occupy themselves happily and creatively at home. If you can develop yourself along these lines now, during pregnancy, you'll be supplying yourself with the tools of occupational therapy as a house-bound mother. "I never tried painting before the baby came, but now I can't wait to get him back to sleep. The hours of the day just fly," one woman told me. Some women find that unless their brains are busy, they feel as if life is over. For them, a college or college extension course while the baby is very small is a good solution to plan for. If you are that type, register for school before the baby comes. Pick a subject, like English literature, that requires a lot of home reading assignments.

If you're an outside person who likes movies, museums, good restaurants, the theater, my recommendation is that you satiate yourself with these pleasures now, during pregnancy. That should tide you over the first months, until the baby is old enough to stay with a baby-sitter or come along with you.

You may find that your feelings about taking vacations from the baby have changed once you've become emotionally attached to him. It's sensible to leave room for this possibility when you're discussing vacations for after the baby comes. I hope both you and your husband will follow *your* feelings and not his. If you feel comfortable about leaving the baby and have competent help at home, you may decide to take a few days off. It's important to do what you both want, first as a mother and then as a couple, and not what other people advise or say is right or wrong.

The most fashion-conscious woman can change remarkably once the babies start to come. The figure she fought so hard to get no longer seems so important to maintain. Husbands often like the new homebody image, but sometimes they object. This is not the woman they married! As a marriage counselor, I hope that if these are your husband's feelings, he will feel free to express them.

Difficult marital problems start when the young husband abdicates to maternity. He gives up on his wife as a sex partner and begins to relate to her as a mother figure. To prevent this regretful situation, frank communication of mutual feelings is vitally important. As he expresses his needs, try to respond to his feelings as well as countering with your own.

On the other hand, a husband's sexual interest, in my experience, is not really in his wife's movie-star image and geishalike behavior even when he believes it is. New fathers soon find themselves responding to their wives' dedication and sincere efforts to be good mothers. If your husband has some superficial values now, the realities of family life with a new baby are guaranteed to help him grow up.

I hope your answer to question 7—"Will I get bored at home?"—is *yes*. Unless they're creative artists—musicians, painters, poets, or writers —most people do. Getting involved in creative homemaking, finding women friends in the neighborhood, becoming active in community affairs are all ways of making the early motherhood years meaningful and enjoyable. No one is more misdirected than the young housewife and mother who feels that her life is without meaning or value, who cannot wait to get back to an office job where she will be doing something "important." It's a sad commentary on the priorities in our society that motherhood and home life are so unappreciated, that a woman can say, "I'm almost embarrassed to admit that all I want to do is stay home with the baby."

Are you afraid you'll become exhausted if you have to get up at night to feed the baby? Most of us operate in a fairly mechanical way. We eat three times a day and go to sleep around the same time each night. A fortunate few of us eat when we're hungry and sleep when we're tired. If you're one of the self-regulators, you won't have trouble with infant feeding. During pregnancy is the time to see if you can let down a bit on the instilled rigidities of a lifetime and become a more natural animal. It will help you get through the first few months, when you'll be tending and feeding the baby every few hours.

Later along, suggestions are made for getting help with baby care. The important thing, I believe, is to want help and reach out for it. Ingenuity in thinking up ways others can participate, and assertiveness in asking them to, are extremely good qualities to develop.

Many women express regret because of what they did or didn't accomplish in raising their first baby. Most often, they will specify the mistakes they made in infant feeding. There were things they were afraid to try, other things that went wrong because of insecurity. Here is the opportunity to reach your goals in motherhood the second time around. If you already have a baby, you are way ahead of the rest of the readers. You *know* which way you want to go

SETTING UP YOUR OWN SUPPORT SYSTEM

When we begin a new life role, all of us need mothering—even new mothers. The major reason for the widespread unhappiness in the first months with a new baby, for the frequency of infant-feeding problems, and for the many tragic postpartum breakdowns that plague young families is the lack of mothering support for the inexperienced mother. She usually has to learn her skills by trial and error, essentially alone.

In other societies, older women who are experienced mothers (usually members of the family or close friends) step in to teach the practical skills to young couples when they marry. In the United States, we are raised to value independence so highly that we have become a nation of isolated individuals and couples. We often live far away from our families and place of birth and feel like strangers in our new communities.

Some young people are finding new ways to replace the supports of the traditional extended family. Sometimes a few couples live together, sharing domestic responsibilities and child care. Others live in larger groups called communes—small communities based on common interests and beliefs. For most people, individual solutions still must be found to help young women move into motherhood.

I recommend that you do everything you can to set up a solid support system to help you with mothering and infant feeding before the baby comes.

First, let us look at some of the supports that are commonly tried. These are expensive, self-defeating, and rarely work.

1. *Staying in the hospital.* A number of doctors report that some women don't want to shorten the time they spend in the hospital after giving birth, despite skyrocketing hospital costs, myriad rules and regulations, tasteless food and bossy nurses, because they are afraid to go home and be alone with the new baby. Sometimes mothers with other young children say they need to extend their hospital stay in order to get enough rest. Some women feel, after the average three-day hospital stay, that they still aren't physically and emotionally ready to take on new motherhood plus housekeeping responsibilities, socializing, and all the normal aspects of adult married life. Instead, they want to rest and be taken care of, to have plenty of time to get to know the baby.

The sad fact is that many breast-feeding women whose milk comes in nicely in the hospital wean the baby within days after hospital discharge.

They become overwhelmed with household responsibilities, scared, and agitated soon after being left alone with the baby.

Sometimes a doctor will recommend staying in the hospital when he knows that a mother is frightened and there is no help at home. But this solution is exorbitantly expensive, and only postpones the inevitable briefly. There are better ways.

2. *Hiring a baby nurse.* This alternative, also not inexpensive, sounds as if it would be a helpful bridge between getting full-time care in the hospital and being on your own. However, it has been found to be a poor solution for most people, unless they have had a cesarean and really need nursing help at home. Most other women report that the presence of a trained baby nurse at home made them *less self-confident* and *more dependent,* and full of problems and fears when she left. Those who attempt to use the period to try their own wings often find themselves engaged in a struggle of will with the nurse. One woman wryly recalls, "We kept fighting about whether the window should be half up or half down in the baby's room." Who knows better, after all, the inexperienced mother or the highly qualified baby nurse? In this case, the mother fired the nurse a week early and got her husband to help out instead.

3. *Hiring domestic help after the baby comes.* This is often a good solution, though it does not work well unless the domestic is a warm-hearted, motherly person who is easy to relate to. New mothers feel very ignorant and vulnerable to criticism. They find it more difficult than usual to relate to a stranger in the house. Besides, few young Americans have experience in supervising domestic help and getting things done to suit them.

More helpful than the day domestic is an experienced, responsible housekeeper who will live in and take full responsibility for running the house, including caring for the other children and doing the marketing and laundry. A good housekeeper hired well before the new baby comes, so she can become part of the family, certainly can be a big help. But this solution is prohibitively expensive for most people, and such competent help is hard to find even for those who can afford it. And one important element still is missing—emotional support for the new mother.

Here are better solutions, which properly support the inexperienced infant feeder as she establishes a relationship with her baby·

4. *Mothering the mother.* The best help, it has been found, is the one most commonly available—the grandmother. In many other cultures, the grandmother moves in with the new family and takes over household responsibilities and the care of the recuperating new mother. If she has a good relationship with her daughter or daughter-in-law, the special plus is that she also loves, coddles, and mothers the mother, which is exactly the emotional food to make maternal juices flow.

In the ideal situation, the new mother learns her skills under her mother's approving, confident eye. The grandmother follows her daughter's cues about what to do around the house, helping her take over again as she is ready. The ideal grandmother selflessly shares her expertise and opinions without imposing her own standards or style of mothering. If she can call upon her empathy—remembering when she was first learning how to be a mother—this won't be hard to do.

Sisters also do nicely at this task, providing there is no rivalry or bossiness. And an experienced, understanding friend will fill the role well. In yogic childbirth, the *sevadar* (helper) stays with the young couple for forty days, which seems like a very generous amount of time to me!

Many of us have neither a mother nor a sister nor *sevadar*. A good substitute is community sisterhood.

5. *The Neighborhood Mother.* If you're living in a garden project or an apartment house with other young families, it's often possible to find a friendly woman who delights in sharing her mothering expertise over the telephone and at coffee klatches. If you're breast-feeding, look for a neighbor who has successfully breast-fed her babies. Visit the neighborhood park, strike up a conversation in the elevator. People love to talk about their babies and themselves.

"When I came home from the hospital, I didn't know anything. My upstairs neighbor was a lifesaver. Every time I got stuck, I ran up. I really couldn't have managed without her," one woman told me.

If La Leche League has a chapter in your neighborhood and you are planning to breast-feed, find out where they are and attend some meetings before you deliver. Besides providing the opportunity to see babies breast-fed and to ask questions, the League will help you make friends who can help you later. (See Part Three.)

Some communities have Mothers' Centers, Holistic Health Centers, and other facilities that teach mothering and infant feeding. Both breast- and bottle-feeders go to their meetings and classes. These are excellent places for learning and meeting experienced people. Visit while you're pregnant. (Many of these facilities are described in Part Four.) Your local ICEA representative knows all the resources in your neighborhood and will help you find whatever you need.

YOUR HUSBAND'S HELP

Women frequently decide to bottle-feed instead of breast-feed because they want to share infant feeding with their husbands. "He doesn't just want to change diapers," they will say.

You'll find that infant feeding involves a great deal more than giving the bottle or breast and putting a blissful baby down. There is burping, soothing, walking, changing, figuring out what might be the trouble. These activities surrounding the actual feeding take much more time than most people realize, and they can be very lonesome and anxiety-provoking to handle all by yourself.

When your husband is there—walking the baby up and down, talking to him, playing with him, calming him—he is calming you too, providing the most precious memories of your infant-feeding experience. A husband's wholehearted participation can transform a potential nightmare into an adventure.

A most important job for the husband is as social buffer. If you live in a garden project or apartment house where people like to drop in, if your relatives and parents visit unexpectedly, his presence and judgment in handling the social situation are invaluable to secure your privacy and peace of mind.

If you're breast-feeding, your husband is the perfect baby-sitter because you know he'll want to keep the breast-feeding going and will never subvert you by offering a bottle when you are not there, unless there really is an emergency. He will be willing to put the time and effort into playing with the baby and distracting him, whereas a paid baby-sitter often won't.

Contract to Share Responsibility

Before the baby comes, sit down with your husband and talk about how you will feed the baby. This is the time for a very honest communication of feelings. You may be surprised to learn that your husband has negative feelings about breast-feeding. He'll feel a lot better if he can air them and be reassured that he won't be neglected and displaced. He may, on the other hand, be very disappointed if you aren't willing to breast-feed his baby and may interpret your choice as self-centeredness.

Also, he may be surprised to learn that you want him to participate actively, although you both aren't sure exactly how. In many young marriages, this will require a temporary change in priorities. Up till this point, attention has centered on the husband's career and getting ahead. Active participation by your husband means a shift of focus. You and the baby come first, his career and personal needs second. Asserting yourself and getting his agreement, in principle at least, will save misunderstandings and hurt feelings later on.

The most important agreement to make is that you will both continue talking about your feelings after the baby comes. Having someone intimate to talk to about your everyday concerns, who listens to your feelings, is the best possible emotional support in the early months of infant care and feeding. If you can express your negative feelings about motherhood and the baby, discouragement will not overwhelm you. The "child" inside all of us needs to be expressed and accepted when we're under stress. When it isn't, childish feelings may be acted out destructively or be repressed and create depression.

Since you don't know exactly what sort of help will suit you best, it usually isn't possible to make detailed arrangements for shared responsibility beforehand. Each couple will have to work out their own plan of action. Here are some solutions other couples have tried that have worked:

1. Share the night feeding, breast or bottle. That means you pick the baby up when he cries, and change, feed, and burp him for the first feeding that wakes you both from sleep. If the baby needs soothing to fall asleep, that's your husband's job. Or he can do the prefeeding jobs and hand the baby to you in bed to breast-feed, and you can get up and take care of the baby afterward until he falls back to sleep.

2. If you're an edgy, anxious infant feeder, you and your husband can sleep separately during the night. The baby, in a carriage, can be rolled back and forth between two rooms.

In this arrangement, the mother picks the baby up for feeding and changing during the night. After burping him, she leaves the baby, in the carriage, next to her husband's side of the bed. In the living room, or wherever there is available space for an extra bed, she can go easily to sleep (with earplugs if necessary), knowing that her husband will wake her when the baby is ready for the next feeding. Usually, he will get up and change the baby for her first.

What is shared here is the responsibility for listening and deciding when to feed the baby. Some women can be very casual about this. They sleep without anxiety, then reach over and pick the baby up for nursing whenever they hear him cry. But others are more anxious. They want to get the baby used to sleeping all night, particularly after the first few months, and are aiming for a schedule.

If the baby is restless and cries out in his sleep, the light-sleeping mother will be disturbed and tense all night. (Many women change into light sleepers right after childbirth and then sleep like a rock again after their last child leaves home.) Having her husband listen so she can sleep between feedings can be a lifesaver for either a breast-feeder or bottle-feeder who is a light sleeper.

3. Sometimes a woman will ask to be relieved of night feedings regularly. In my experience as a family counselor, this is not usual unless her husband and mother have encouraged her dependency and play on her weaknesses. Most women feel responsible for their babies' care and are convinced they know how to feed them better and more sensitively than anyone else. If a woman is breast-feeding, she knows it's not a good idea to skip any feeding during the first six or seven weeks, while she still is building up her milk supply.

New mothers try very sincerely and know their own limits. Most are under considerable tension as they're learning, and this in itself is exhausting. The most helpful attitude a husband can take about night feedings or any other household responsibility is that his wife, not he, should decide what she needs.

Your Husband as "Confident Parent"

While the woman needs babying and coddling herself in the first weeks after childbirth, a continuation of this "mothering" is not what she wants afterward. What is the most supportive attitude a husband can take after she has recuperated to help her grow more confident in herself as a mother?

The husband can take on the role of "confident parent." Just as parents of adolescents help their growing youngsters to overcome their dependency, so the husband can support his wife's capacities as a mother and respect her authority to make the decisions regarding the baby's care and feeding.

Many feeding decisions will have to be made in the first years. When is it all right to leave the baby with someone else for the evening or for a day's outing? When and how should the baby be weaned from the breast, from the bottle? When should solids begin? What about a pacifier? Should the baby share the parents' bedroom? Until what age? Should the baby always be responded to when he calls or cries? Until what age?

If the husband continues to view his wife's mothering role as the major job in the family while the babies are small, encouraging her and supporting her decisions, he will be solidifying the marital relationship more than he realizes. Both he and his wife will go on to other individual goals later in life, taking turns supporting each other's aspirations. Since there are so many stresses and strains in even the best of marriages, a husband's loyalty and support of his wife as she learns how to be a mother is "money in the bank" emotionally. And, unless you are luckier than most people, the good feelings of your partner are an emotional resource you will be calling on, time and time again, in the many years of family life that follow infant feeding.

Part Three:

GETTING INVOLVED

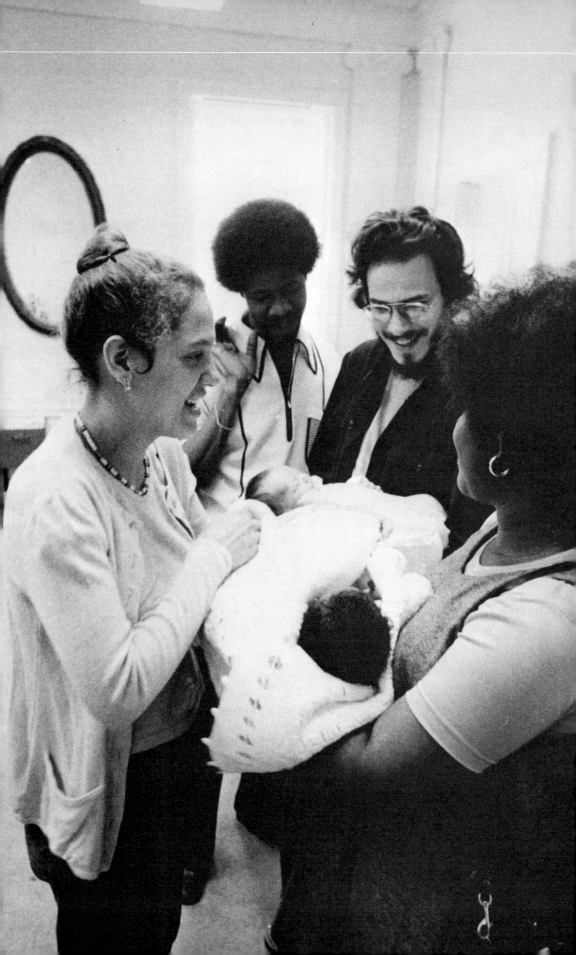

9

Step 1
Tapping Your Key
Community Resources

By now, you have decided whether or not you want natural childbirth. You have selected your feeding method. Your next steps will ensure that you get the help and cooperation you need to carry these choices through and to give you the protection you will need if unforeseen problems make your first choices unfeasible.

Most couples still select the closest doctor and hospital, sign up, and leave all the decisions to the experts. All they do then is pay the bills. Other couples shop like knowledgeable consumers for the least costly service that gives them exactly what they need and want. Rather than rushing to make arrangements as soon as you know you're pregnant, it is wiser to sort out your .preferences, read about the options, and draw up a list of what you want before you commit yourself. There are four important organizations available to help you implement your choices. They know where your options can be found, and their goal is to help you locate them.

These alphabet agencies look strange now, but I hope you will soon become familiar with them and let them help you find the resources you want. Each organization has somewhat different goals, but all are working to improve American childbirth. They cooperate with one another, and the leaders of all of them are the most knowledgeable people in your state about every program that is opening up and every facility that is available. They will help you find family-centered hospital care, home birth, help with breast-feeding, childbearing centers, and special education for infant care and parenting. According to your own special interests, one or more of these groups will give you the help you need.

Couples from the Maternity Center Association preparation classes get reacquainted with their new babies. Some groups go on to postpartum education. (Paco North/Maternity Center Association)

ICEA (International Childbirth Education Association, Inc.)

MAJOR GOAL: Family-centered maternity care.

INTERNATIONAL OFFICE: P.O. Box 20852, Milwaukee, Wisconsin 53220.

LOCAL GUIDANCE: In Appendix I are the names and telephone numbers of province/state ICEA coordinators. They know your local resources and will refer you to health care providers and facilities that are family centered in philosophy and practice.

TO JOIN: Individuals are invited to join ICEA for $12 a year, professionals for $30. Members get one vote, the *ICEA News*, a membership directory, discounts on publications, books, conferences, conventions, and local meetings. Write to: ICEA, Membership Clerk, 195 Waterford Drive, Dayton, Ohio 45459.

In 1960, parents and professionals (both as individuals and groups) formed this organization to promote a better childbearing experience. Members are autonomous, with their own policies and programs. Some are involved with childbirth education (all the prepared childbirth groups discussed in chapter 7 are members of ICEA), while others specialize in education for good infant care and parenting.

Because they're all working together, the members of this international organization are providing outstanding leadership in the childbirth field. They have speakers available, and publish a quarterly for professionals, a newsletter for teachers, a newsletter for group administrators, and a newsletter for the general membership. Members meet locally, at regional conferences, and at international conventions.

ICEA reviews and sells books and publications about childbirth and parenting through its Bookcenter. For information and a free catalogue, write to: P.O. Box 70258, Seattle, Washington 98107, or call 206 –789-4444. Three times a year ICEA publishes *Bookmarks*, a free review of all new published materials (sent on request). The organization's own publications, for the public as well as for members include *Parent's Guide to the Childbearing Year*, *Teacher's Guide*, *Father Participation Guide*, and a *Film and Record Directory* (a list of childbirth films for rent or sale). A free catalogue of all ICEA publications also will be sent if you write to: ICEA Publications Distribution Center, P.O. Box 9306, Midtown Plaza, Rochester, New York 14604.

Although the major work of ICEA is to promote better childbirth and pediatric care by doctors and other professionals, assist existing programs, and help new ones start, the organization also sponsors its own programs. These include assistance with teacher training programs (including self-training for people who live in isolated communities), childbirth and parenting information, and parent-support groups. (Part Four will describe some of these groups for you.)

Call or write your ICEA state coordinator (Appendix I) if you need a referral to a doctor or hospital or if you want parenting education during pregnancy or after the baby comes. You will find these people knowledgeable, responsive, flexible, and eager to help.

NAPSAC (*The National Association of Parents and Professionals for Safe Alternatives in Childbirth*)

GOALS: To bring information on all childbirth alternatives to the public at large.

To bring all birth choices—both in and out of the hospital—into mutual cooperation by providing a forum for communication and cooperation of parents, medical professionals, and childbirth educators.

To refer the public to birth attendants and organizations all over the United States who offer natural-childbirth and family-centered care in hospitals, childbearing centers, and safe home births.

To assist in the establishment of maternity centers, family-centered maternity care in hospitals, and safe home-birth programs.

To provide parents and parents-to-be with the education to help them assume more responsibility for pregnancy, childbirth, infant care, and child rearing.

NATIONAL OFFICE: Marble Hill, Missouri 63764.

LOCAL GUIDANCE: The national office will refer you to doctors, midwives, home-birth organizations, and childbearing centers in your locale.

TO JOIN: To receive their news quarterly, be kept informed of research activities and notified of upcoming programs and publications, and participate or just generally support the organization, send $6 a year to the national office.

NAPSAC is a very new organization. It started in November 1975 as an idea of David and Lee Stewart (childbirth educators in the Bradley method who were active in ICEA) to bring together everyone interested in promoting alternatives to traditional hospital childbirth in the United States.

Dr. Stewart is a professor of geophysics. His wife Lee was a music teacher until their Bradley classes and five children kept her too busy to pursue that career. Their children were all born at home, with David Stewart the only attendant.

Fifteen years ago, when the Stewarts tried to find a natural-childbirth facility that would provide rooming-in for Lee and the baby and permit David's participation in labor and delivery, there was none in their local area. Lee comes from a home-birth farm family. Both she and David felt that medication was dangerous and separation of the mother and baby a poor way to start.

David explains, "It was not our wish to have an unattended birth, but to have a competent attendant. But there never was a doctor or midwife available to come to our home for any of our children's births." So the Stewarts went ahead on their own, with the cooperation of a local obstetrician who agreed to be on call in case of emergency. "We didn't talk about it to other people," says David. "I just caught my babies. Lee pushed them out; I never pulled on any of them. It was an experience incomparable to any other in my life. Many fathers are reluctant to get involved, but I have never known a father who was present once who would ever miss that experience again!"

And their five births were not all uneventful. One baby was born with the cord around his neck ("This happens in 25 percent of births," says David. "I just slipped it off.") and two were posterior presentations. The small tears repaired themselves. "The obstetrician wasn't worried about stitching them up," says Lee, "and there were no sexual problems afterward."

Lee wanted her older children close by during subsequent births, so they would not feel excluded. As she had anticipated, it meant a great deal to the Stewart children. "Our children absolutely would be upset if they were not included," she says. David also feels that having siblings present is more important than we realize. "Rivalry is an artifact of the way we give birth in the United States. A child accepts his mother, and if he sees the baby as part of the mother, he will accept the baby, too. . . . Our kids fight, but they're not rivals. Another child simply is not a threat."

The Stewarts don't recommend that other people follow their example of do-it-yourself childbirth, but, they say, "Many people still have the same dilemma we faced fifteen years ago. We are compiling a good list of birth attendants from all over the country, adding to it every day, but many people still can't find anyone in their area to help them. People have a choice of negatives—unattended home births or a hospital that will not cooperate with the idea of a natural, humane birth. They have to do some soul searching and decide which kind of risk they want to accept. We give people credit for the ability to make their own decisions and handle their own lives.

"Half our Bradley couples give birth at home, the other half in the hospital," they continue. "One of our main services in NAPSAC is to provide the information that will help people make up their own minds. We refer them to. ICEA for help in finding family-centered maternity services, to home-birth services that educate them to manage their own home births, if necessary, and provide criteria for selecting qualified home-birth assistants. We offer a reading list and the findings of our own research institute."

Under the direction of Dr. Lewis E. Mehl, NAPSAC sponsors The Institute for Childbirth and Family Research, at 2522 Dana Street, Berkeley, California 94704. The Institute will send you a list of its research papers, which include findings on complications in home births, outcomes of early hospital discharge, and management of complications of home delivery.

"Freedom of choice without opportunity is no choice at all," decided the Stewarts in 1975, so they organized the first national NAPSAC conference to explore alternatives in childbirth. More than five hundred people, mostly childbirth experts, came to that meeting and agreed on the need for an organization. The second annual convention had eleven hundred people, about a thousand of whom are now NAPSAC members. More than two thousand are expected at their 1978 convention, where the topic is "Compulsory Hospitalization or Freedom of Choice in Childbirth?"

The Stewarts also plan regional conferences that will give members an opportunity to meet and communicate. They are printing a list of all the alternative services they have located and have just published the papers of their second conference. Research Director Mehl is now setting up a model homelike childbearing center in Berkeley that is much like the Maternity Center's model in New York. It is called The Family Health Center, at 2522 Dana Street, and the telephone number is 415–849–3665.

NAPSAC is expanding so rapidly you will have to keep in touch with the organization to remain up to date about all their new activities. From their new home in Marble Hill, Missouri, the Stewarts will direct you to an alternative birth center or a home-birth assistant, if there is one in your locality. Since laws about the legality of home birth differ from state to state and there is professional as well as legal risk for doctors or nurse-midwives who come to your home, you may find it very difficult to get qualified help. However, with all childbirth experts working so closely together, with the unique focus and enthusiasm of NAPSAC and the Stewarts, who knows? Perhaps by the time you read this, a qualified, well-trained birthing assistant will be available in your own backyard. And, David Stewart assures you, "NAPSAC will always be on the frontier."

ASPO (American Society for Psycho-Prophylaxis in Obstetrics)

MAJOR GOAL: To promote the development and acceptance of psycho-prophylactic childbirth preparation (Lamaze method).

National office: 1523 L Street NW, Washington D.C. 20005; tel: 202-783-7050

LOCAL GUIDANCE: In Appendix II are the addresses of your state ASPO chapters. When you write, they will refer you to your local ASPO resources —chapter leaders, teachers, doctors, and cooperating hospitals. Many local ASPO chapters regularly survey their neighborhood hospitals and are up to date about their regulations and facilities. If you want rooming-in, unlimited husband visits, sibling visits, early discharge, ASPO can let you know if the possibilities exist in your immediate neighborhood or if you will have to travel elsewhere.

ASPO also is starting many special support and educational programs—for teenagers, for couples after the baby comes, exercise classes for new mothers, and the like. If a particular kind of service is available in your area, even if ASPO does not offer it, the organization will know about it and refer you to the right place. Like ICEA (of which it is a member), ASPO has developed its own national network of services and also works cooperatively and closely with other childbirth and parent organizations.

To JOIN: Doctors, parents, and childbirth teachers all can join ASPO. The regional or state coordinator (see Appendix II) will refer you to your local membership chairperson. Fees vary according to locale, with part going back to the national organization. Approximate fees are: teachers, $60 a year; doctors, $35; parents, $7.50; single, $5.

In 1951, French obstetrician Fernand Lamaze traveled to Russia. He was greatly impressed by what he saw of Russian childbirth practices and introduced many of the principles into his own practice in Paris, adding a fast-breathing technique and several other modifications.

In 1959, a young American woman, Marjorie Karmel, wrote a book called *Thank You, Dr. Lamaze* about her excellent experience giving birth with his method in Paris. She had trouble finding similar help here for the birth of her second child, wrote an article about it in a national magazine, and drew attention to the Lamaze method and the need for training classes in the United States.

Physiotherapist Elisabeth Bing, still a distinguished Lamaze teacher in New York, arranged to meet Karmel and set up the original classes. In 1960, she and medical professionals founded ASPO. In an effort to eliminate the unfavorable public attitude toward "natural childbirth," they introduced the term "prepared childbirth."

Since that small beginning, ASPO has publicized and gained acceptance for prepared childbirth all over the United States, trained thousands of teachers and more than a million couples. In 1977, it expected to have 3200 teachers teaching 288,000 couples the Lamaze method. It is a growing, lively organization, with three active branches—parents, professionals, and physicians. Proud of its accomplishments and its leadership position, ASPO maintains the highest standards, works cooperatively with other childbirth organizations, and is interested in innovative programs. Its teachers and chapter leaders try to organize groups in response to their communities' needs, and are aware of every private and public service available. You can call on them with your ideas, your requests for service or for referrals to doctors, hospitals, and support groups before and after the baby comes.

La Leche League, International

MAJOR GOAL: Good mothering through breast-feeding.

LOCAL GUIDANCE: Write to the national office, 9616 Minneapolis Avenue, Franklin Park, Illinois 60131, or call 312-455-7730. You will be referred to your local La Leche leader, who knows the local obstetricians and pediatricians in your area, particularly those who support breast-feeding mothers. They also know which hospitals encourage breast-feeding through rooming-in, nurse encouragement, extra feeding time, etc. La Leche leaders, like the ICEA and ASPO people in your area, know exactly what is happening in childbirth in your neighborhood— which new resources are opening up, which support groups are being organized. They work closely with nutritionists, childbirth educators, hospital nurses, obstetricians, and midwives in the area. I have found that whenever there is a particularly difficult personal or professional problem to solve, the local La Leche leader in my neighborhood is the person to call.

In 1956, in Franklin Park, Illinois, seven nursing mothers and their friends formed the La Leche (Spanish for "The Milk") League to learn about breast-feeding from one another, share experiences, and offer mutual support. By 1960, there were 20 La Leche groups; by 1969, there were 775 in all fifty states. Now there are about 2500 groups in the United States and more in other countries. La Leche League reaches more than a million people a year through group meetings, correspondence, telephone conversations (women in any area where there are no meetings available can call experienced leaders for personal telephone help), and their journal.

The basic La Leche manual, (see Bibliography), prepared by the original group of mothers, has sold more than 600,000 copies in the present edition. Informative leaflets, pamphlets, and books are available from the national office about prenatal care and childbirth, breast-feeding, child care and the family, the League itself, nutrition, and the psychological aspects of mothering.

Despite the phenomenal success and growth of La Leche, not everyone you speak to will support or praise it. In fact, many professionals—including doctors and childbirth educators—will have something negative to say: "They are fanatic." "They make the mother feel guilty if she stops nursing." "They are so persistent I have to pry them off a case." "They never admit that nursing is contraindicated for the mother or the baby."

The League has very good reasons to be so dogged about educating mothers to continue breast-feeding despite difficulties. It has had to counteract a great deal of anti-breast-feeding propaganda in a culture where the practice has almost disappeared. The League is popular where it counts—among young, inexperienced breast-feeders who need all the help they can get.

If you're at all interested in breast-feeding, I recommend that you meet your local La Leche group months *before* delivery. Use their help in locating the best pediatrician to help you manage a breast-feeding baby. The socialization experience itself is invaluable. Women you meet at La Leche will give you a warm welcome, show off their babies, and radiate their obvious delight in being mothers. They might give you conflicting advice about how to prepare your nipples or which cream is best to use, but their friendship and concern will see you through the first weeks and months of breast-feeding, which are the hardest times.

Step 2
Finding Your Birth Assistant

For most American women, the obstetrician is the birth assistant of choice. His training and expertise in handling the abnormalities of labor have lowered the maternal death rate in this country until it is among the lowest in the world. As Dr. Stanley James points out, "Mortality has fallen so dramatically that women aren't afraid of dying or undue pain in childbirth anymore. We live a much freer life."

There are other kinds of doctors delivering babies in America. Some are older, experienced general practitioners who maintain the kind of family practice that includes delivering babies in the hospital or, less frequently, at home. Their patients wouldn't have it another way.

In Chicago, which has a long, successful history of home births attended by young doctors and medical students through the Chicago Homebirth Service (now closed), a group of physicians recently formed The American College of Home Obstetrics "to cooperate with families who choose to give birth in the home, to learn from and teach each other the art of safe supervision of home births." Their headquarters at 664 North Michigan Avenue, Suite 600, will refer you to a trained physician, who will assist in your home birth, if one of their members lives in your area. (NAPSAC also has a small listing of physicians who perform home or office deliveries.)

After many years of mistrust, more women are turning to midwives as birthing assistants and, in a rapidly growing renewal, more than one hundred settings have trained nurse-midwives delivering babies, under the supervision of or with the back-up of obstetricians.

Your choice of a birth assistant should be determined by three things: his or her expertise, philosophy, and personality. I believe that in normal childbirth, as in psychotherapy, the quality of the relationship is much more important for a successful outcome than the formal credentials of the helping person. It is the practical experience of the birth attendant and the rapport established with the mother that make for a successful and safe birth. Many natural childbirths are failing because of poor communication and bad "vibes" between the normal, low-risk patient and her highly certified and qualified doctor—who might be the perfect person to help her if she had special medical problems. The personalities of the two people most involved have to mesh in an atmosphere of easy acceptance and communication. *Mutual* trust is very important. You must trust your birth attendant, to be sure, but he also must trust in and have respect for you.

INTERVIEWING THE OBSTETRICIAN

If you intend to have an obstetrician as birth attendant, you will need to know how to find one with whom you can establish the kind of relationship I've just described.

Your childbirth teacher, one of the "key community resources," recently delivered friends, or a pediatrician can recommend obstetricians to you. Hospitals will give you only a formal list, with no personal description. Even with personal recommendations, it's still *your* job to interview obstetricians so you can find the one you'll work with best.

If you have a chronic physical problem, like heart trouble or diabetes, it's a good idea to find a specially qualified obstetrician through your local medical association, medical center, or the American College of Obstetricians and Gynecologists. You also can check if an obstetrician is board-certified (with special advanced training) by writing to the American College of Obstetricians and Gynecologists, 1 East Wacker Drive, Chicago, Illinois 60601. Similarly, you can check whether a general practitioner is certified in family practice (has maintained continuing education with postgraduate study) by writing to the American Academy of Family Physicians, Volker Boulevard at Brookside Boulevard, Kansas City, Missouri 64112. Don't be dazzled by credentials, however. They are important, but no matter how well qualified the doctor is medically, you still have to be able to get along with and trust him or her in a very personal situation.

If you're expecting a normal childbirth, I recommend that you meet a number of doctors, unless you are truly enthusiastic about the first one you interview. Unless a physical examination is included, there should be no cost for this first meeting.

Dr. Robert Fitzgerald, chief of the Doctor's Division of Long Island ASPO, suggests, "Find out exactly his philosophy and whether he meets your specific needs. Patients have a right to know what they're getting. Make an organized list and discuss it with the doctor. Ask him to make an exception for you if you have a specific need. Be stubborn, open— and don't be afraid. The doctor will refer you elsewhere if he doesn't have the conviction to carry through on your demands."

The Bradley natural-childbirth people also advise that prospective patients prepare an "options list" before they interview a doctor. In their preparatory "early bird" class, they even role-play the interview in advance. Their suggestion is that the first office visit be by the couple rather than the woman alone, "so your demands will be taken seriously."

What if you aren't sure what your demands really are? Doctors differ in opinion about IVs, monitors, episiotomies, and "prepping." Some accept them as the usual regulations, but would just as soon forego them if the hospital agrees. Others believe that some of these rules—particularly for routine use of the electronic monitor—are very important. Patients' feelings likewise range from indifference to outrage about each of these procedures.

What you need is a good "fit" between your point of view and the doctor's, an impression that a relationship will be easy to establish. If you can talk comfortably with the doctor the first time you meet, you're off to a good start.

Here is a brief checklist to help you evaluate how you are relating to the doctor personally. Since you'll be living with that relationship for nine months, it's important that it begins on a positive foundation. As you're talking, does he seem to you: persuasive, sincere, overwhelming, bossy, sarcastic, too formal, too personal, too easygoing to rely on? Does he seem to understand and feel sympathetic to your philosophy of childbirth and to your life-style? Do you find it easy to ask questions and present your options list? Do you trust what he says and have a positive feeling toward him? "See if you can relate to and trust him as a *person*," suggests Dr. Fitzgerald.

Remember that you will be very vulnerable once you're in the middle of labor and delivery. Then the doctor can support you by his presence and his attitude, or he can ignore you or leave you on your own. The gentleness of his internal examinations, his manner and procedures in delivery, will matter very much.

Here are some questions to ask him about his routine practices.

1. Does he routinely do episiotomies?
2. In natural childbirth, does he hand the baby to you on the delivery table?
3. If you're awake and aware, will you have the baby in the recovery room?
4. Will he arrange for you to move around in labor or will you have to lie down?
5. What kind of monitoring will he do of the baby's heartbeat?
6. Do you have to be strapped down on the delivery table and put your knees in stirrups?

Ask about any hospital routine—IVs, enema, shaving—and regulation—private rooming-in, early discharge—that particularly interests you, and find out his ideas and feelings about them. What are his views on drugs and anesthesia during childbirth? Do most of his patients end up with pain relief? What proportion of them breast-feed?

Here are some examples of patient-obstetrician relationships that were off to a poor start, and went downhill from there. It would have been better, at the beginning, to find a more sympathetic obstetrician.

"I knew he didn't like me from the beginning. He thought I was a kook because I was Jewish and didn't want to circumcise the baby. He kidded me about it all through the pregnancy, every time I visited, and I saw it bothered him. On the delivery table, when I had a girl, he laughed and said, 'I think I'll circumcise her.' By then I hated him so much I wouldn't go back for the six-week checkup."

"It made me nervous, the stiff way he had of calling me Mrs. C. while he was examining my private parts. Finally, I asked him to call me Susan and he agreed. But he added, 'Just don't call me George!'"

Keep in mind that it's the obstetrician who has the ultimate authority to discharge you from the hospital, while it's the pediatrician who must agree to take on responsibility for the baby's discharge. In the best situations, the obstetrician and pediatrician know each other and have worked together frequently. "The doctor can act as your agent and mediator," says Dr. Fitzgerald. "It's what benefits the patient, not the hospital or the doctor, that's important." Some hospitals are inflexible about their policies, and the doctor will find it difficult to implement any unusual demands. In that case, is he associated with another hospital that has less rigid policies?

The quality of your relationship should improve in the months before the baby comes. You will have many questions and the best doctor is the one who is accessible and relaxed about answering them. What will happen if he's delayed en route to the hospital? How will you know exactly when to start out for the hospital? Who will deliver the baby if he's on vacation? Can you meet that other doctor before your due date?

If you seem to have more than normal anxiety about giving birth, the doctor may refer you for psychological help. If your marital relationship is under a strain because of your pregnancy, counseling with an expert may be indicated. Ordinary concerns do arise and should be discussed with the obstetrician. For example, doctors differ in their recommendations about continuing normal sexual intercourse in pregnancy, but all should be willing to talk about sex openly, without being prodded so that you feel embarrassed.

In my opinion, a conscientious obstetrician will refer you to the La Leche League for support and help if you plan to breast-feed, except in the few cases where he knows your pediatrician provides special breast-feeding education. In many neighborhoods, the inexperienced, first-time breast-feeder finds herself isolated, without another woman to consult, and such a contact can make all the difference in her success in breast-feeding. Pregnancy is the time to make these contacts, not when you're tied down with a new baby.

A conscientious doctor will raise the question also of your nutrition in pregnancy. If he has a rigid attitude about weight gain, and pooh-poohs the idea of nutritional supplements when you're interested in them, he is far behind the times. What you want is an open-minded, flexible attitude; this is more important than a wide knowledge of nutrition.

In this day of group practices, shiny new offices, expensive fees, hurried interviews, and full waiting rooms, it's important to select an obstetrician carefully if you are to get the support and help you need. Rather than seeking out the most fashionable doctor in town, why don't you look for a friendly doctor who will take the time to develop a personal relationship? If possible, find one like the Bradley doctor on Long Island who told me, "For a good relationship, more time is needed in the office. Women are full of questions, and they call up a lot. But I enjoy the questions. It makes my job more interesting."

THE CASE FOR THE QUALIFIED MIDWIFE

"We are the experts in the care of the normal woman during pregnancy and birth," says Mary Ross, a nurse-midwife from the Maternity Center Association's Childbearing Center in New York. "The obstetrician deals with any complication that may arise throughout pregnancy, labor, or birth."

This understanding of the qualified midwife's expertise has been accepted by doctors as well as nurse-midwives. In 1971, and again in 1975, the official organizations of both groups issued a joint statement agreeing that "there are defects in the availability and quality of maternity care, not confined to any particular social class," and that these defects could best be corrected by the cooperative efforts of a team approach. "In such medically-directed teams," they concluded, "qualified nurse-midwives may assume responsibility for the complete care and management of uncomplicated maternity patients."

"One of the things we nurse-midwives are trying to do is provide prenatal, labor, delivery, and postpartum care for the essentially normal family. This enables obstetricians to have more time for complicated cases," says nurse-midwife Irene Sandvold of Washington, D. C., who is an advisor in the Family Health Division of the Pan-American Health Organization, World Health Organization of the United Nations.

Only a few years ago, not many of us knew exactly what a midwife is or where she might be found, but today, "We have to avoid advertising because of the terrible influx," reports Judith Roehner, a nurse-midwife at Downstate Hospital in Brooklyn, New York. "Why do women come? They're seeking a flexible, naturally oriented, open-minded kind of care, rather than a disease orientation. They feel more at ease with another woman, and want the continuous support and counseling we make available twenty-four hours a day. Our midwives teach childbirth classes, preparation for breast-feeding, and family planning."

For many women, delivery by a nurse-midwife in a special unit of a large medical center seems the perfect answer. All the things they hate most about hospital delivery are absent: "prepping," routine IVs, and electronic monitoring; having to stay in bed during labor; having to move into another room to deliver; routine episiotomy; being separated from the baby. And all the advantages they dream about are offered freely: freedom for the husband to participate fully; instantaneous medical backup, with the latest technology, in case of complications; a

Leboyer-like delivery with dim lights and a warm bath; help with breast-feeding and baby care; and, most important, a well-trained, friendly professional who stays with them right through labor and delivery.

For other women, however, the absence of a male obstetrician feels like second-class care. Even though they expect nothing to go wrong, they would rather be in the hands of a specialist.

And for a third group, the hospital setting makes childbirth too much of a "medical event." They see the nurse-midwife as a starched shadow of the warm-hearted woman who comes into your home, shares your life-style, attends the delivery, and mothers the family. One woman told me, "Here in California we want to do things our own way." She and her friends are assisted by a lay midwife, who doesn't have professional certification, but does have plenty of practical experience, obstetrical and hospital backup in case of emergencies, is willing to come into their homes, and is very inexpensive.

How qualified can a lay midwife be? For that matter, how qualified is the nurse-midwife? Is is really safe to have anyone but a doctor deliver your baby? You'll be as surprised as I was when I found out the answers.

Brief History of Midwifery

Midwifery is one of the world's oldest professions, described in the earlier books of the Old Testament. Midwives were accepted members of the social structures of ancient Greece and Rome.

The first American midwife was the wife of a doctor and came over on the *Mayflower*. Midwives dominated obstetrics in America until the nineteenth century. Then their role was taken over by doctors, who considered these women's work anachronistic and unqualified. Soon midwives were legislated into oblivion.

Many Americans still associate midwifery with the Dark Ages, even though midwives deliver 80 percent of the world's babies, including the majority in such technologically advanced countries as England, Sweden, Germany, and The Netherlands. Midwifery also has been in continual practice in some parts of the South and Southwest of our country, despite medical antagonism and public distrust in other sections of the country. "Granny midwives" have been working independently in poor rural areas, some self-taught, some trained by local doctors, and some trained abroad.

The first American training school for midwives was in New York. It was open from 1915 to 1935, and during that time a number of other small schools, in other parts of the country, opened and closed.

The great heroine of American midwifery, Mary Breckenridge, decided to devote her life to the health care of children in remote areas. A nurse who lost her husband and children in an accident, she went to England to study midwifery, then came back with some English nurse-midwives and opened The Frontier Nursing Service in an inaccessible, hilly section of Kentucky, where the people were impoverished and completely without qualified medical services.

Her Frontier Nursing Service began as a home service only. Today there is a modern hospital and six outpost clinics staffed by qualified

Almost fifty years ago the Frontier Nursing Service proved that safe homebirths are possible even in the poorest surroundings. (Hans Knopf/ © 1975 by Frontier Nursing Service)

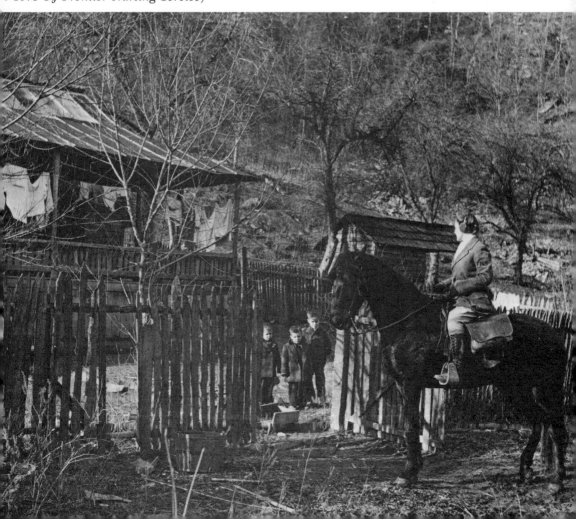

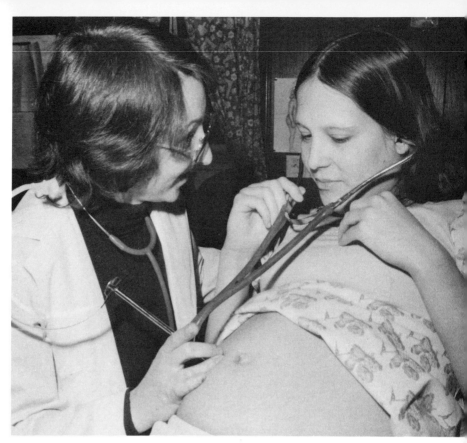

Today the same personal care is available from the Frontier Nursing Service midwife, but up-to-date hospital care is also available when necessary. (Gabrielle Beasley/ © 1977 by Frontier Nursing Service)

nurses and nurse-midwives who furnish home and clinic care to some four hundred families each in the area. They use all modern equipment, including radio direction from doctors at the central hospital when needed, and travel in jeeps (it used to be on horseback) to visit families and deliver babies at home. In their first ten thousand deliveries, the Frontier nurse-midwives have kept their maternal mortality to one-third of national and state levels. Their patients could be termed "high-risk" because of their poverty and malnourishment, yet in the past twenty years they have not lost a mother. Their nurse-midwifery training school, started in 1939–40 (when the original English staff returned home to help in the war effort), has the distinction of having trained a large proportion of the nurse-midwives who work in the United States to-day.

Nurse-midwives were trained even earlier in New York. In 1931–32, the Maternity Center Association (described in chapter 7) sponsored a school, which delivered many New York babies in poor sections until 1958–59. Then the school was transferred to a local hospital and the home-birth service was closed, "because of the high-risk factors associated with home birth in the inner city."

Other nurse-midwifery training centers opened in other parts of the country, most with home-birth services. Today there are seventeen centers where a registered nurse can get midwifery training in the United States for deliveries in hospitals, and there are over one hundred hospitals and a few childbearing centers where she is permitted to practice.

Nurse-Midwifery Today

For referrals: write or call The American College of Nurse Midwives, 1012 14th Street NW, Washington, D. C. 20005, 202–347-5445. They will send you a list of hospitals near you that have nurse-midwife units and can inform you about any childbearing centers, private practices, and independent practices in your locale.

In order to be admitted to a training program today, nurses must have a bachelor's degree with a major in nursing, a heavy concentration in science and math, a license as a registered nurse, one year's experience in public health and one year in-patient hospital experience, as well as personal and professional references.

By the time training is completed eighteen months to two years later, the nurse-midwife will have participated in about 120 deliveries and have more experience in normal childbirth than the average general practitioner. She rapidly accumulates so much experience thereafter, working full time with normal births, that she soon knows more about managing normal pregnancies and childbirths than the average obstetrician.

Nurse-midwives were available only to poor people, in home and hospital care, until quite recently. Their services opened up to other women mainly because women clamored for them once they heard of their excellence and their superior outcomes (their statistics are much better than the national average statistics for hospital deliveries).

Many obstetricians still resist referring middle-class patients to nurse-midwives. Doris Olson, president of ICEA, reports, "They still use nurse-midwives as obstetrical aids and delivery-room nurses." However, there is a slow but sure trend toward acceptance and appreciation of their training and expertise, and a fuller use of their services. Many state governments are passing or beginning to consider licensing bills that would allow nurse-midwives to work independently of hospitals and doctors. Most importantly, childbearing women are beginning to know about them, trust them, and select them as birth assistants.

You usually will find the nurse-midwife in a large hospital as a member of the medical team. In facilities specializing in advanced intervention, they remain an oasis of natural practice. Sometimes they're provided with special homelike facilities, but often they deliver babies in ordinary labor rooms that have nothing special about them except more freedom, warmth, and extra attention for the patient.

In some hospitals, they deliver up to 50 percent of the babies. They screen out some kinds of high-risk situations in advance—a mother with high blood pressure or diabetes, for example—but they deliver twins or breech babies, since all the safeguards of the hospital are right there in case of complication. They do not perform cesarean sections.

Both clinic and private patients see nurse-midwives today. If you're a clinic patient, call the nurse-midwife unit to find out which days you can see a midwife. If you're coming in privately, you can visit in advance, meet the midwives, and make your private financial arrangements. Fees are fixed (like the obstetricians') for pregnancy care, birth, and the postpartum period. The midwife's fee is almost as high as the obstetrician's, but since early discharge is almost automatic, you will save on the hospital bill.

Private patients are traveling considerable distances to get to midwives, who are willing to accommodate anyone who will make the trip to the hospital. There is a restriction on travel time for home visits, however, so patients coming from distances longer than one-half hour make their own pediatric and visiting-nurse arrangements for follow-up care in the days after delivery. Then they come back to the hospital for regular checkups, and regular telephone service, twenty-four hours a day, is available for all patients. For many people, the most important advantage is the knowledge that they can rely on the midwife's dedication to natural childbirth. She will protect them from unnecessary interventions, yet provide them if and when they become necessary.

Certified nurse-midwives also are delivering babies in "childbearing centers" (there are nine at the time of this writing, with many more in the planning stage), homelike, out-of-hospital settings that are described in the next chapter. The American College of Nurse Midwives and

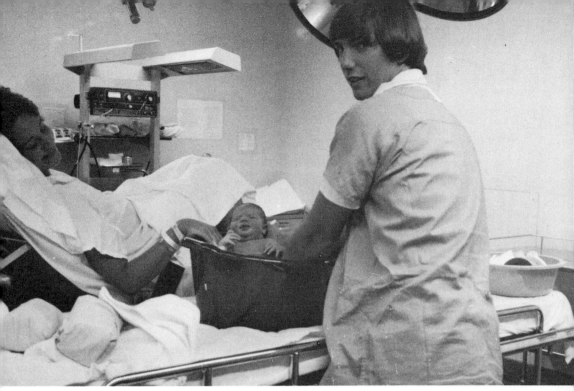

Natural childbirth with a nurse-midwife is available in some of our up-to-date teaching hospitals like Downstate Medical Center in Brooklyn, New York. (Nurse-Midwifery Associates, Downstate Medical Center, Brooklyn, N.Y.)

Out-of-hospital childbearing centers are increasing in number for normal, low-risk deliveries. Here husband and midwife work together at the big moment. (Alison Ehrlich Wachstein, from Pregnant Moments, Morgan & Morgan, *1978)*

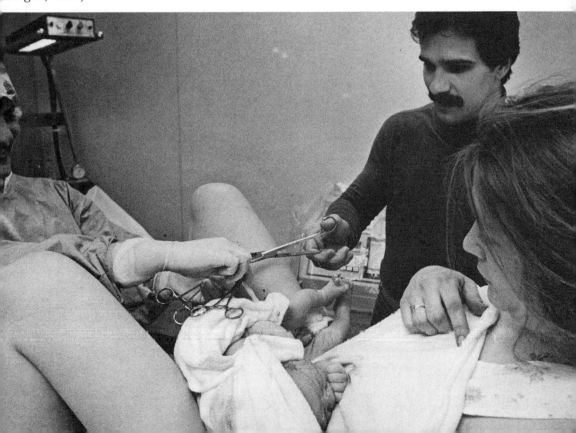

NAPSAC both keep up to date on these new developments, and will let you know if there is a childbearing center available in your own community, perhaps nearer than the closest nurse-midwifery unit in a hospital.

A number of intrepid nurse-midwives have developed independent home-birth practices, with privately arranged obstetrical and hospital backup. One of these, which is serving as a model for others throughout the country, is Maternity Center Associates, Ltd., of Bethesda, Maryland.

A Model Nurse-Midwifery Prenatal and Home-Birth Service

Maternity Center Associates began in October 1975. Two young nurse-midwives, graduates of Georgetown University, wanted to practice on their own in the community. Maryland law specifies that nurse-midwives may not practice independently or collect fees, so they formed a corporation and hired two "backup physicians" to give "medical direction" (these men are actively involved and available for emergencies). The midwives then proceeded to see patients and deliver babies. Doctors who work with them are called "medical consultants" and their patients are called "clients" because they are normal, healthy people. The midwives will not deliver a baby at any risk, including twins or breech position, and screen constantly for continued normalcy during the pregnancy.

The association has grown and expanded rapidly, though the women do not solicit patients or advertise, are occasionally harassed by the local medical society, and are opposed by most local obstetricians. At this writing, they have hired an additional nurse-midwife to work with them on a rotating basis, and six extra doctors as "hospital backups," who will admit their clients to local hospitals as their private patients in case there is any problem during labor or delivery.

Since starting, the nurse-midwives have been delivering twenty to twenty-five mothers a month, with a superior record of safety. About 15 percent of their clients have had to be hospitalized, most for cephalopelvic disproportion (the baby's head is too big to get through), which often cannot be predicted during pregnancy.

They have a sliding scale and a regular fee, $550, which is a lot less than the usual doctor-plus-hospital fee private patients pay. A few insurance companies cover their service, but Blue Cross and Blue Shield do not. The amount of service clients get for their money is astonishing.

First, they have a pleasant, modern clinic, with play facilities for older children. In the initial orientation, the parents agree to make all required home preparation, provide pediatric backup, attend childbirth preparation class and meetings of HOME (a national home-birth organization that prepares parents for home birth). Parents also have to provide a birth assistant—a nurse or a friend who is knowledgeable about basic nursing procedures. The association will hire someone for them if necessary, for $50 to $100. This assistant is there to help the nurse-midwife with the delivery.

The nurse-midwives feel that "If women want home births, the professionals providing prenatal care have to practice improved, if not superior, prenatal care." They see their clients very frequently throughout pregnancy, establish warm and close relationships with them, and work hard to straighten out any nurse-client relationship problem before delivery so the client will be equally comfortable with all three midwives. Clients fill out their own charts and review lab work with their midwives. "We see ourselves as technical advisers. We are not trying to be their fathers and mothers."

Two weeks before delivery, a midwife visits the home, to make sure she will be able to find her way when the time comes, and to meet the family. The client, meanwhile, has made arrangements for emergency hospitalization if necessary and posts the telephone number of the local ambulance service. "If a mother does not do these things, we will not consider her for a home birth. The whole business of having your baby at home is that you have to be very responsible, yourself, for the care you are getting," says Marion McCartney, vice-president and co-founder of the service, who herself is the mother of four youngsters, all born in the hospital by cesarean section.

Janet Epstein, president and co-founder of the association, describes the home atmosphere during birth: "We are guests in the client's home, and we don't take over. We don't wear uniforms. Instead we wear blue jeans and shirts that say 'Happy Baby Home Delivery Service,' which helps keep things casual and optimistic. We don't do anything routinely —not shaves, enemas, episiotomies, or anything like that. Such things are done only as needed. . . . We do try to offer a lot of options. In so far as the situation remains normal, our clients can do and suggest almost anything. We have had clients who want to use a variety of different positions in labor, others who want to handle their babies in a particular way. . . We will use some of Leboyer's methods [see chapter 11], as little or as much as the client wants. We will turn out lights, turn on lights, bathe, not bathe. It really doesn't matter to us. We consider ourselves hired experts—there to help and to monitor things so that everything goes well."

Marion McCartney adds, "One of the unique things about our service is that about half our babies are delivered by the baby's father rather than by the nurse-midwife."

After delivery, the nurse-midwife remains with the mother for about two hours and puts the required silver nitrate in the baby's eyes. The pediatrician then takes over responsibility for the baby while the midwives remain on call, twenty-four hours a day, if anything comes up for the mother. Clients are seen for checkups at two weeks, six weeks, six months, and one year after the birth. They can go, free, to postpartum groups run by a psychiatric nurse practitioner, who explores their family relationships and the stresses of having a new baby around. Marion McCartney says, "We are absolutely delighted with the results we've gotten so far, and most of our clients, I think, are better than satisfied." Janet Epstein says, "These are normal, thinking people—a joy to deal with."

Services like this are only beginning to develop, but they promise to grow into an important childbirth option in the future. They are inexpensive, safe, beautifully structured, richly human resources. What seems to be required for the nurse-midwives interested in starting such services, in addition to professional quality and expertise, is the willingness to shoulder great responsibility, the ability to withstand considerable legal and other pressure, and the acceptance with aplomb of the legal description of their service as a "business corporation."

Private Practice

As always, there are a few independent souls who prefer to work on their own. These are fully qualified nurse-midwives who make their own arrangements for medical backup, emergency transportation and hospitalization, and will deliver your baby at home. The legality of this practice is at issue in some states and there is considerable pressure against it, both from the professional nurse-midwife organization and medical groups, so you will have considerable difficulty locating a certified nurse-midwife who will deliver your baby at home on her own. NAPSAC will refer you to one if they know of her existence, and you can also inquire from one of the home-birth organizations described in the next chapter.

The Lay Midwife

To find a lay midwife: Write to NAPSAC, Marble Hill, Missouri 63764, or The National Midwife Association, P.O. Box 163, Princeton, New Jersey 08540

Since there no standards yet for the practice of lay midwifery, you have to take the great responsibility of checking the lay-midwife's credentials and her record in home births. Sometimes a lay midwife is very well educated and qualified. She may not be licensed because of a legal liability such as foreign training. More often she is a person who has gained the experience without the professional credentials, but some are unprepared, inexperienced, even charlatans.

Many lay midwives are very concerned about establishing good standards of practice, and they have banded together to form an organization that is working toward this end. They would agree with Dr. Gene Cranch, assistant director of the Maternity Center Association, who is very concerned about the spread of home births with unqualified assistants, or, even more dangerous, the do-it-yourself home birth. Says Dr. Cranch, "There are many lay midwives who are very skilled and who know their limitations, when it's safe to deliver at home and when to get help. What worries me are the ones who have done only a few births and think they are experts."

Here are the views of one outstanding American lay midwife, Nancy Mills of California, who delivers babies at home and in hospitals, trains other lay midwives, directs a clinic at which obstetric residents train, and is hard at work trying to establish realistic standards of training that lay midwives will be able to afford. These remarks are taken from her addresses to the first NAPSAC convention and the recent convention of nurse-midwives in New York:

> Lay midwives have been practicing in Texas and Appalachia for about thirty-five years. They are not illiterate, and their usual educational level is high school, although not all are graduates. None has had formal training, but many report being trained by

physicians. Most want more training and are aware of their limitations. In communities where they are available, the lay midwife usually is chosen over professionals, including doctors and nurse-midwives, because mothers feel they receive better care in their homes.

It is going in the direction that most babies will be delivered by midwives. In the area I am in, it could be up to two hours' drive to the town with the nearest available obstetrical care. The women are just not coming in. Ten percent of births are at home, many of them unattended. At the clinic, we're getting all economic levels and a number of religious groups, including Jehovah's Witnesses, Mormons, and Seventh Day Adventists.

Many of the doctors in Sonoma County say, "If we could get rid of Nancy Mills we wouldn't have this problem." Well, I really disagree. They can get rid of me, but then they will just have to get out there and do it themselves. People want to control their experience. Some of them have had a hospital experience. Fifty percent are requesting a home birth. We do not propose it, we do not encourage it. . . . Our philosophy is that a woman has a right to a choice.

II

Step 3
Finding Your Birth Setting

Some people learn the hard way how important it is to have a good setting for childbirth: "I always felt I wanted my babies with me. Mother and baby need each other right from birth. But I learned the hard way how important it is to differentiate between hospitals and what they give you. In my second delivery, they separated my husband from me, and I panicked. The third was so much easier. My husband is so attached to the children. I think the way I give birth has something to do with it."

BONDING: WHY YOUR CHOICE MATTERS

The place you choose to give birth helps to shape your whole experience of childbirth. You may be staying in a hospital for only three days, less than that in an alternative setting, or you may never leave home at all to have your baby. But these brief days and hours are unforgettable, and the comfort and security you feel then can strongly affect how you begin motherhood, how you relate to the baby, and your husband's feelings, too.

Just as animals find the safest, most secure, most comfortable environment before settling in to give birth, so should we feel it our biological right to search out an optimal setting for our deliveries. Sometimes, no matter how well you choose, your childbirth experience will be disappointing, difficult, even painful. But since the atmosphere can affect your feelings, and your feelings affect your ability to relax and be spontaneous, you can see that it's all-important to arrange a setting that will work best for you.

In the first hours after a normal, undrugged childbirth, the mother and baby, when given the opportunity for unhurried, unsupervised physical contact and privacy, will "bond"—become emotionally attached and tuned in to each other in a pleasurable, easy, natural way.

Drs. Klaus and Kennel, in *Maternal-Infant Bonding* (see Bibliography), describe the biologically-determined-specific sequence of behavior in which human mothers engage when they first meet their infants:

> Most mothers *touch* their infants in a pattern of behavior that begins with fingertip touching of the infant's extremities and proceeds in 4–8 minutes to massaging, stroking and encompassing palm contact with the trunk. . . . The mother makes *eye contact* with the baby in the "en face" position [she swivels her neck to look him full in the face]. . . . She speaks to the baby in a *high-pitched voice*, which fits in with the infant's sensitive auditory perception. In a process called *entrainment* the newborn moves in rhythm to his mother's voice. . . . The mother is the *time-giver*, reestablishing the baby's body rhythm, first established *in utero*, which is interrupted by being born. The *odor* of the mother affects the baby, and it is possible that the olfactory system may be found to play an essential part in attachment to the mother. The *heat* of the mother's body keeps the baby warm, and contact with her and with her *breast milk* builds his resistance to infection and offers immunity to certain illness.

The process is reciprocal. The mother is affected by the baby's voice and odor. The eye contact is mutually rewarding. The flow of hormones that make her feel motherly is initiated by closeness to the baby, and finally "mother and baby become locked in a sustained reciprocal system."

Here is how one mother described the bonding with her infant in a home birth: "You just want to hold the baby in your arms, and when you do, everything feels complete. You get very attached to the baby when she's inside, and when you realize she's out, safe and in your arms, it's wonderful!"

This same mother described her suffering when the normal bonding process was interfered with in an earlier hospital delivery: "The first feelings were awful, frustrating. They just held my baby up for a second and whisked him away. After I went through the whole thing, they took away the reward! I had a terrible hunger for him in my room and kept thinking I could hear him in the nursery, crying for me. . . . Once I was in the car with the baby, I really let go. I felt as if my chest were cracking open, and I sobbed and sobbed. My husband asked me what was wrong and I said,

'Nothing, I'm just happy!' I counted the baby's fingers and toes and said, 'He's mine now.' "

If a mother is heavily sedated or feeling ill after childbirth, she may not have the physical or emotional energy to make contact with the baby. But if childbirth has been normal, she will feel a need to hold, make eye contact with, and stroke the baby. The effects of keeping these feelings bottled up turn possible feelings of pleasure and fulfillment into bitterness and disappointment that can have long-range consequences for her later attitude toward the baby.

There is a considerable amount of data showing that close contact between mother and child immediately after birth is extremely important for the future closeness of the baby to *both* parents. Those early sensitive moments have long-lasting effects on both parents' feelings of acceptance of and empathy with the newborn. The father who has access to the new baby—and who can hold, fondle, and make eye contact with him—can become as "engaged" with the baby as the mother.

Emotional stress—not just physical separation—can interfere with bonding. Stress caused by a recent move to a new home, marital infidelity or unhappiness, the death of a close friend or relative, or the loss of a previous child, can all interfere with a mother's normal ability to relate to and respond to her baby.

In a setting that allows it, the mother begins breast-feeding within a few minutes after the baby's birth. This strengthens her motherly feelings (breast-feeding stimulates the flow of hormones that increase motherliness) and provides the baby with all the physical advantages of immunity and relaxed respiration that go along with breast-feeding.

A home setting is not necessarily best for the breast-feeding experience. Some women need the support and encouragement of hospital nurses:

"I felt like a little baby myself—so well taken care of. The nurses were so considerate and patient. They were proud of me for nursing, pampered me, and the milk just flowed in. I needed that pampering—too much, I guess. Once I got back home, I felt lonely and scared, and when my nipples got sore, I gave up nursing."

But other women report that the hospital interfered with both bonding and breast-feeding: "I felt embarrassed nursing the baby in front of the other women. They weren't nursing and weren't fumbling around like me. At night when they brought the baby in and woke me up, I was afraid I'd wake the other women up. I was relieved to get back to my home and privacy."

By and large, being alone with the baby when learning how to breast-feed has been found to be most conducive to both bonding and successful breast-feeding. You do need to forego visits from friends and relatives while you're in a rooming-in situation, but your husband can stay as long as he likes. The three of you will be so busy adoring one another you won't miss other company at all!

Instead of considering these issues, women are still selecting hospitals because they're big and famous. Before you choose a large medical center with a neonatal clinic and complete blood bank, measure your likelihood of needing these services against the advantages of a family-centered setting.

Another frequent reason for selecting a hospital is that your doctor is affiliated with it: "I figure I have a good doctor. I'll let him handle me, tell me what to do and where to go." Before following blindly, measure the importance of that relationship against what you may be giving up in terms of intimacy with your baby in the first days after birth.

An increasingly common reason for choosing a less desirable setting is resistance to traveling for prenatal checkups and particularly for delivery: "It's such a hassle to get into the city. I'm afraid of the traffic when I'm going to the hospital to have the baby." By pretiming and mapping the route to a better setting that will accept you, you can arrange to get there in plenty of time, particularly for a first or second baby. Check carefully what to look for so you'll know when to start out. Don't assume you are ineligible for any setting that interests you. Many will accept anyone for service who is willing to make the trip, and some people come from hours away.

Because they're new and unfamiliar, many women still believe that any out-of-hospital alternative can't be as safe as a hospital. Although statistics are limited because these services are quite new, the opposite may turn out to be the case. Their outcomes are remarkably successful, safe, and uneventful medically. Of course, high-risk patients are screened out, but if your pregnancy is healthy and your labor and delivery are likely to be normal and uneventful, natural childbirth may be more successful in an alternative setting than in a traditional hospital. Going the established route, to the local hospital, is no guarantee that you will not be upset and disappointed by your childbirth experience.

Many women are, which is why alternatives are being developed. What happens to you depends to a great extent on physical events, but your psychological relaxation in the setting of your choice is also a large factor in a normal childbirth.

Some women believe that staying home is the only way to feel safe and secure in childbirth. Sometimes a mother-to-be has had so much unhappy exposure to hospitals with sick family members that she is emotionally allergic to the hospital environment and would be better off in an alternative setting. If you feel this way, find a good birth assistant to help you, and make good, safe arrangements for a home birth instead of trying to overcome your morbid fear of hospitals.

A good rule in childbirth, as in life, is "Let your head guide your feelings." That means find out what your feelings are, respect them, but act on them with good judgment.

IS A BIG HOSPITAL BETTER FOR YOU?

"Where would I take my wife to have a baby today? To a large training hospital that delivers more than two thousand babies a year and has the latest equipment," says Dr. Mike Finster of Columbia Presbyterian Hospital in New York. "That's where we went, of course."

Dr. Finster, and many other knowledgeable people, is sure the impersonality and discomforts of a large setting are worthwhile tradeoffs for the top care they believe such hospitals provide. Here is what Dr. Sprague Gardiner, recent president of the American College of Obstetrics and Gynecology, has to say: "I think it's pretty well shown that unless a hospital has one thousand deliveries or more per year, it can't afford to support the personnel and equipment needed to provide really quality care."

A 1967 national study by the American College of Obstetricians and Gynecologists (ACOG) revealed that most deficiencies in maternity care were associated with small hospital size, few deliveries a year and lack of teaching facilities. They made the following recommendations for three levels of hospital care in childbirth:

1. *Perinatal centers* with high-risk maternity clinics, newborn intensive-care nurseries, round-the-clock laboratories and blood banks, genetic counseling, all the advanced equipment for monitoring and the

like—that deliver a minimum of five thousand babies a year—for the 10 percent of women at high risk. (Women are considered to be at high risk today not only if they have a physical condition that might affect their pregnancy, but also if they are unwed, separated, divorced, under twenty, over thirty-five, poverty-stricken, or subject to any unusual stress.)

2. *Quality-care hospitals* with intensive-care units that deliver two thousand or more babies a year for most women.

3. *Smaller hospitals* that deliver a minimum of five hundred babies a year and can arrange transport for either the mother or baby to a center with more facilities when necessary—for women who live in remote rural areas.

In another interpretation of the same statistics, the American Foundation for Maternal and Child Health points out that the larger obstetric services have a greater rate of maternal and infant deaths. They conclude that while, undoubtedly, some of these deaths result from the fact that there is a greater rate of high-risk mothers delivering babies in larger teaching hospitals, it also is likely that there is a greater tendency to intervene in these institutions, especially in order to provide learning opportunities for students and residents, and that this also contributes to the poorer maternal and infant outcome.

Doctors and administrators at smaller hospitals, which are faced with the threat of being closed through the implementation of this ACOG "regionalization" proposal, contend that they are the ones providing the supportive, flexible atmosphere so necessary to women in natural childbirth. Perhaps to attract patients, these hospitals offer family-centered innovations like private twenty-four-hour rooming-in and birthing rooms. Their staffs believe that they know the limitations of their facilities for high-risk situations, and also know very well when and how to transfer patients who need more advanced equipment and care to nearby medical centers.

Keep in mind that extraordinary services are needed in only one in ten hospital deliveries, while supportive surroundings are psychologically indispensable for all natural childbirths. Perhaps family-centered maternity units offering natural childbirth will be an option in all large hospitals of the future. Meanwhile, my recommendation is to check the reputation for safety and flexibility of the hospitals in your area before you decide what hospital is best for you.

From the patient's point of view, hospitals differ from one another for a different set of reasons—their atmosphere and their regulations. Some are overwhelming, impersonal, and rigid places with decor to match. Others seem like a second home for their personnel, but not their patients. Still others provide cordial and attentive surroundings, nicely decorated and homey.

Some hospitals have stringent regulations—limited visiting hours, routinely used electronic monitors, separation of the mother and baby for up to twenty-four hours after birth. Others are flexible about what equipment must be used in labor and delivery, provide special services for natural-childbirth and breast-feeding mothers, and are willing to accommodate the attending doctor's practices and special requests for a patient.

In many hospitals, the doctor has more power to bend the rules than the patient is aware of. When he says something is "against hospital policy," he may mean simply that the hospital prefers it to be done a certain way and he doesn't choose to ask for an exception for you. Some doctors are amenable to making special requests if you ask for them, and these exceptions don't necessarily present problems either for hospital personnel or administration.

"I see myself as a mediator and agent between the patient and the hospital. Hospitals should be more flexible and make hospital deliveries more attractive," says Dr. Robert Fitzgerald of Long Island ASPO. "We try to be flexible and bend the rules," says nurse-childbirth educator Gladys Lipkin of North Shore Hospital on Long Island.

One way of arranging for a satisfactory hospital experience is to ask your local doctor to work as your mediator and agent with the local hospital. If you do not care to be an exception, however, it may be wiser to find a hospital with the features you want, even if it is farther from home, and use its help to locate an affiliated doctor you can relate to.

FINDING THE FAMILY-CENTERED HOSPITAL

Family-centered care means a childbirth experience that includes the supportive involvement of your husband or other companion of choice. Depending on the setting, it can mean: provision for your husband's involvement in labor and delivery; active breast-feeding support;

birthing rooms and rooming-in facilities; and early discharge. To find hospitals that offer some or all of these family-centered features:

1. *Contact your ICEA or ASPO state coordinator* for a hospital referral. Let them know which family-centered features interest you most so they can refer you properly.

2. *Local La Leche and childbirth leaders* know even more about local color—atmosphere, possible room for exceptions, attitude toward breast-feeding mothers. They also can put you in touch with other women who recently delivered at local facilities, or know a lot about good facilities somewhat farther away.

3. *Ask the hospital directly.* Rules and regulations change frequently in response to consumer demands. For the most up-to-date information, call the maternity supervisor of your local hospital and ask the following questions (adapted from the ASPO hospital survey forms):

- Is my husband allowed in the labor room if he has taken a course of preparation? Is he allowed in the delivery room? Is he required to leave if I have any medication at all, if I have anesthesia? If my doctor agrees, can my husband stay if I need a cesarean? Can a different companion accompany me if he or she is prepared by a course?

- Is there rooming-in with the baby? Part of the time or twenty-four hours a day? Is it possible to have a private room for rooming-in?

- If there is no rooming-in, how many times a day is the baby brought in for feeding? Are there extra times if I breast-feed? (More frequent feeding is important for stimulation of the breasts, to help the milk come in.)

- Will the nurse help me breast-feed? Is there an evening hour set aside for my husband to come and learn how to feed and care for the baby with me if I bottle-feed?

- What is the visiting policy? If I have rooming-in, can my husband come as often and stay as long as he likes? Can my older children visit?

- Is it possible to leave earlier than the usual three days if my obstetrician and pediatrician agree that the baby and I are ready to go home?

SOME COMMON FAMILY-CENTERED FEATURES

Some innovative hospitals are offering one or more of the following (the ICEA will direct you to them):

Birthing Rooms

A major improvement, offered in some family-centered hospitals, is a homelike sitting-bedroom for labor and delivery that spares mothers the unnecessary stress of being transferred to an operating-room setting when they are ready to deliver. Both obstetricians and nurse-midwives associated with the hospital can use the birthing room.

At Smithtown General Hospital on Long Island, local PEP Lamaze mothers helped plan and implement the birthing room. An administrator says, "We didn't want to overlook the needs and personal con-

Birthing rooms are not only "cozy," they spare the mother the stress of moving from labor room to operating room at the peak of labor. (Morris Warman/New York Medical College, Flower & Fifth Avenue Hospitals)

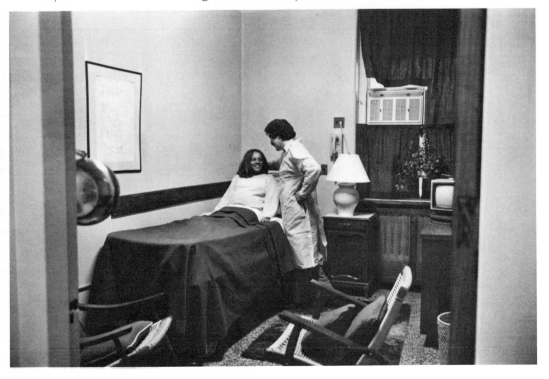

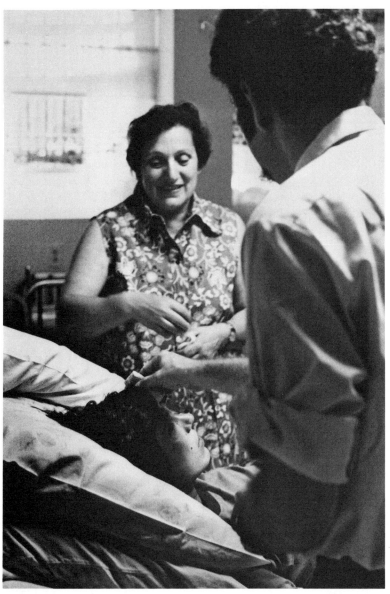

An innovative feature of some hospitals allows the supportive presence during labor and delivery of a husband, grandmother, or other companion of the mother's choice. (Ed Lettau/Maternity Center Association)

cerns of the low-risk patient or impose obstetrical technology on her. Any low-risk, natural-childbirth mother and her obstetrician can use the room. They are transferred to the delivery room for C-section or any other obstetrical intervention. We do require exterior fetal monitoring, but it's on a cart, so the mother can move around, sit in a chair, or lie down. There is a couch for her husband to rest on, too.

"The bed is a high, single hospital bed, with automatic lift and lowering. There is no other equipment kept in the room until the time of delivery, when an instrument cart comes in. We can dim the lights if the doctor and mother request it.

"Mothers have demanded this facility, and they're delighted with it. There is no extra fee, and more doctors, especially the younger ones, are using it all the time."

Smithtown General is an example of a smaller facility that is responding to the needs of the community as expressed through local childbirth and parent groups. Soon they plan to institute partial rooming-in and sibling visitation. As one innovation succeeds, the next one is tried more enthusiastically.

Midwifery Care and Delivery

More large hospitals are adding midwife delivery services, for both private and clinic patients.

In these large training hospitals, one section will offer the most advanced obstetrical techniques and another will have the low-key natural-childbirth unit, usually with nurse-midwives in attendance. Since obstetrical and pediatric backup are available, mothers don't necessarily have to be "low-risk." For example, some of these services will deliver breech or twin babies.

Nurse-midwife Theresa Dundero's description of her unit at Albert Einstein Hospital in New York City offers a good example of how these services operate. In some hospitals, facilities are more lavish; in others, they are smaller and less agreeable.

"At Einstein, the midwives utilize labor rooms, but these are decorated like a bed-sitting room, with bed, lounge, and chair. The mother is not restricted to the bed, and we don't monitor routinely. We use the monitor in special situations—if the heartbeat is slow or if there is staining.

"Only a small number of our mothers need to be transferred to the delivery room. If they are transferred, they are wheeled in on their own bed. We have only a bulblike syringe for suctioning the baby, but that's usually enough. Other suctioning and resuscitation equipment is in the delivery room. Since most mothers take no medication and are given the baby for nursing directly after birth, we have not had to use medication to stop bleeding.

"We do screen out women with cardiac conditions, diabetes, or high blood pressure, but other kinds of 'high risks'—like twins or breech—can be handled. Anyone willing to make the trip can come, but we can't make the usual two home visits if they live more than a half-hour away by car. We do have twenty-four-hour telephone service. We ask mothers to call us if they're bleeding, have fever, or abdominal pain.

"Most women go home in twelve to twenty-four hours. Our staff pediatrician examines the baby first, and we have found that most local pediatricians are willing to make home visits on the second and third days. We also teach mothers to take care of the immediate newborn, to check for jaundice, and see her and the baby at home on the second and third days.

"Our mothers use the Bradley and Lamaze methods. All of them are breast-feeders. They take their preparatory classes outside, but we recommend books and offer educational material. We see mothers every four weeks at first, then every two, and, at the end, every week. If a mother is "late" on her due date, we do lab testing first—such as urine tests. Then, at forty-three weeks, an obstetrician is brought in and the oxytocin challenge test is recommended."

This hospital alternative already is available at nineteen hospitals in municipal New York. The ICEA can tell you if it exists in a hospital in your area. It is safe, and less expensive than being delivered in other parts of the hospital, partly because of early discharge. If you're sure you want natural childbirth, and would feel most secure delivering in a modern hospital with every advanced facility right there, "just in case," you might look into a nurse-midwife hospital delivery.

Sibling Visitation

More and more family-centered hospitals are offering this innovation—which is one mothers of young children have been asking for for many years. Surprisingly, it is becoming much less difficult to arrange.

In the company of a responsible adult, a child of any age is allowed to visit his or her mother and the new baby at a special hour during the day. The mother sees her other youngsters in a special visiting room and accompanies them to the infant nursery to see the baby. In some hospitals, the children are allowed even closer to the baby, but this is less usual because of the fear of transmitting colds.

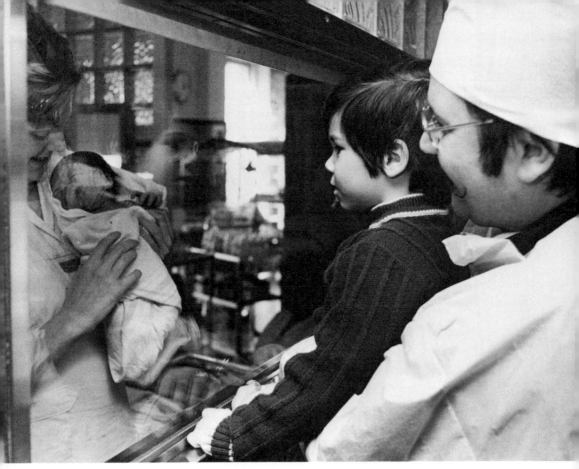

More and more hospitals are allowing siblings to visit, an option worth requesting. (Edward J. Bogard, Jr./Elizabeth General Hospital, Elizabeth, N.J.)

"It keeps the mothers happy. They love it," I've been told. It's also enormously reassuring to other little children to see where their mother is, to know that she's well and will be home again soon.

MORE CONTROVERSIAL OPTIONS

Other family-centered options are more uncommon and controversial. These include sibling participation at birth, twenty-four-hour private rooming-in, early discharge, and Leboyer delivery. Despite the possible emotional advantages for mothers and babies, there are possible adverse factors that must be taken into consideration. Here are the pros and cons.

Sibling Participation in Childbirth

One reason some couples are having home births is that they want the whole family to be together. They feel it's important to get the new sibling relationship off to the best possible start by having the other children observe and even participate in the birth, reassuring and supporting the mother. Instead of having to accept a little stranger into the home after three days, the toddler or older child identifies with his beloved mother's feelings of joy when the baby comes. Pointing to the cooperation and mutual support of the "Walton" type of family in America's past, these advocates feel that by restoring family closeness at childbirth, we can avoid the rivalry and insecurity that so many youngsters suffer today.

Many others are appalled at the idea of "inflicting" childbirth on a young child, who can so easily misunderstand and misinterpret his or her mother's cries and facial expressions of stress and pain during childbirth. This is a personal response no less deserving of respect and attention than the other.

Experts differ on this subject, just like everyone else. A mother's feelings about having her other children present, to observe and interact with her, during childbirth, should be the determining factor.

Here is the reaction of one two-and-a-half-year-old, as reported in a local paper: "Nathan was excited and looked on with a giant smile. He stayed glued in his rocking chair. He simply said, 'Oh baby! Baby!' as his brother was born. The next day he wanted to share his cookies with his new brother. Now he beams proudly whenever he sees him. The parents said, 'We'd certainly do it again.'"

Twenty-four-Hour Rooming-In

Twenty-four-hour rooming-in usually starts when the mother and baby come down from the recovery room together. They stay together in the same room until she is discharged, unless the baby needs some special medical attention. He is in a bassinet at her side, and she learns from the nurse how to hold, feed, and change him. Everything is quite relaxed. Her husband can visit any time during the day and evening and participate in baby care, but no other visitor is allowed into the room.

Childbirth experts support this arrangement enthusiastically. As Ruth Lubic, director of Maternity Center Association, says, "It provides the best education for the mother—unlimited contact with the infant from birth."

Here are some common objections to this procedure. First: "Maybe the mother will get dizzy and drop the baby." I believe this fear is generated by the malpractice specter that is haunting doctors and hospitals.

After natural undrugged childbirth, most women nap or rest briefly, but then are ecstatic, full of pep, and delighted to be with their baby. Second: "The baby needs a constant trained observer. The mother might miss a sign of distress." Since nurses are always visiting the rooms to observe the babies themselves and to teach mothers how to observe their babies' breathing, sucking, and sleeping habits, "rooming-in babies" tend to get more attention than babies in nurseries. Rooming-in floors are distinguishable from nursery floors as soon as you step off the elevators. You never hear a baby cry.

Partial rooming-in, which some hospitals offer, is not the same experience at all. The nurses are in charge, not the mother. The baby is wheeled in and out to accommodate rounds, visiting hours, cleaning people, and so on. Mothers usually must share a room, which makes for a lot of socialization, not a sense of privacy. Night breast-feedings become brief and furtive, because the other mothers are asleep, and the mother is frustrated afterward because she never knows how the baby acted after being fed. Sometimes the nurse will decide to skip the night breast-feeding and not wake the mother because she thinks the patient needs the night's rest. What is gained is one night's sleep, but what is lost is the mother's self-confidence that she can totally satisfy the baby.

The most important disadvantage of partial rooming-in is that it usually begins twelve or more hours after birth. Thus mothers and babies lose the irreplaceable opportunity to bond at the prime biological and psychological time.

Early Discharge

Frequently, after just one day of rooming-in, many mothers feel ready to go home. Hospitals are very expensive—more than $100 a day—children cannot visit, and the mother feels well enough to begin to miss her home surroundings. Rarely is the mother permitted to follow her own inclinations.

In response to persistent consumer demand, however, many hospitals are beginning to bend or officially change their policies about early discharge. When the mother, obstetrician, and pediatrician all want it, these hospitals will agree—usually with the stipulations that the mother sign a special release form and that the baby be seen daily at home by a pediatrician or other qualified observer.

Many people, even childbirth teachers, still believe that hospitals are legally bound to keep babies three days for routine tests. But, as childbirth educators Jim and Jane Pittenger found out through personal experience, "Hospitals are not jails; you *can* sign yourself out!" After the delivery of one of their babies, they did just that, finding a pediatrician to help them at home. Then they carefully wrote to their obstetrician, explaining the reasons for their action. By the next delivery, they had established such a good relationship with the doctor that he made the early-discharge arrangements with the hospitals for them.

"It's not the law that keeps babies in hospitals," I learned from obstetrician Robert Fitzgerald. "It's up to the pediatrician." All the neighborhood pediatricians I asked in a telephone survey assured me that routine testing of babies can be done in the office as well as in the hospital, and that they would have no objection to making home visits after early discharge.

"Doctors who advocate early discharge have the percentages very much in their favor," the director of the Ambulatory Pediatric Service of the University of Wisconsin Medical School in Madison, Dr. Catherine De Angelis, told me. "There is no harm is sending babies home early if risk situations are carefully excluded, and there is an assurance of continuity of care. An intelligent mother can be trained to observe the baby for signs of distress. . . . However, if the mother is still recuperating and doesn't have the proper help at home, it might be better to have her stay for a few days where she can rest and have trained people to help her if necessary."

I discussed early discharge with neonatologist Dr. Lawrence Gartner of Albert Einstein Hospital in New York, who said, "In general, yes, it's safe for mothers to take babies home after twelve hours. But it requires careful screening—of the mother's history and the baby's delivery and postdelivery history. The child should be carefully screened in the hospital and there should be a well-structured and organized home-visiting program. The baby should be seen each day for the first three days.

"Mothers rarely recognize jaundice," he pointed out, "because the baby looks so well. But they can learn to look out for the baby who is not feeling well, who has fever, rash, or other evidence of infection. A trained visiting nurse also could handle the newborn observation. This is the common practice in other parts of the world, where the nurse accompanies the mother home."

VISITING NURSES

The visiting nurse no longer will routinely come to your home to show you how to bathe the baby, as she did for your mother. But she will come if you need help, and usually her service is free in maternal-child situations. Most Visiting Nurse Association referrals come from doctors, hospitals, and other agencies, and the nurses will come only if there is a supervising doctor on the case.

If your pediatrician wants the visiting nurse to act as his trained observer, you can call and give his name and telephone number to the Visiting Nurse Association in your area. The nurse will come to your home the same day you call, or the next day at the latest, and will repeat the call if either she or the doctor thinks it is necessary. You can get the telephone number of your local Visiting Nurse Association from your local directory, or your local hospital will give it to you.

Rooming-in, early discharge, and follow-up by your doctor or visiting nurse often can be arranged if you're persistent. For many women, the combination of twenty-four-hour rooming-in and early discharge is the most satisfying childbirth arrangement possible. The feeling is that the entire hospital and community are working for you, providing the support and warm personal care you need, allowing you the freedom to decide when you are well enough to go home and take care of the baby yourself.

LEBOYER CHILDBIRTH

French doctor Frederick Leboyer concluded, after years of obstetrical practice and research, that our common delivery-room practices damage newborn babies physically and emotionally. He believes that more sensitive procedures can help create happy, optimistic human beings. After his book was published abroad and extensively in America a few years ago, Leboyer traveled extensively to discuss his delivery-room procedures, which make the transition from the womb to the world a pleasant rather than an abrupt and painful experience. A film of one of his deliveries was shown on American television, and he spoke at many public meetings of childbirth experts and obstetricians. For the past few years there has been a slowly growing interest in his method here. American research has begun to explore the effects of his delivery procedures on early mother-child bonding and the later development of babies. While many doctors are not too interested in modifying their delivery-room techniques, slowly it is becoming easier to arrange for a Leboyer-like childbirth.

The core of the method is avoiding sensations that will jar the new-born baby. Leboyer used soft lighting, a warm bath, and gentle massage after the delivery to evoke womblike sensations and ease the transition into life. Modifications can include soft music and dispensing with bath and massage, according to the setting, the philosophy of the birth assistant, and the preferences of the parents.

Leboyer's observations about "birth trauma" under ordinary hospital delivery conditions are supported by some psychological findings. As far back as sixty years ago, psychoanalyst Otto Rank developed a whole psychological theory connecting later psychological temperament with birth experience. Arthur Janov is finding that many patients recall upsetting birth experiences in the course of primal therapy. Stanislav Grof's recent work in LSD therapy substantiates earlier psychiatric theory about the importance of womb and birth experience on later development.

Most obstetricians aren't taking any of this "psychological stuff" too seriously. Many equate turning off the bright lights in the delivery room with the Dark Ages, and worry about whether it's really possible to maintain a constantly warm temperature in the baby's bath. Dr. David Kliot, an obstetrician at the Brookdale Hospital Medical Center in Brooklyn, who has had considerable experience with Leboyer births feels differently: "We have stayed with the techniques because we feel that's what makes childbirth safe. . . . The low ambient light is not a critical factor, it just takes away from the hospital atmosphere. Bright lights can be shocking to the baby. Leboyer babies retain their alertness for an hour after birth. They lift their heads and move around. They love the bath."

Every Leboyer doctor and midwife works somewhat differently. Dr. Kliot's application of the Leboyer method would satisfy the objection of childbirth educators and parents who feel that Leboyer seems to value his massage and bath techniques more than the mother's breast as a comfort for the just-born baby.

"Right after birth, I put the baby face down on the mother's abdomen if the heart rate is good, turn out the lights, and ask for quiet. The babies don't cry, their heart rates go right up. On the mother's skin, the baby's temperature is retained, with no cold stress. I don't believe that waiting to do the cord clamping until pulsation ceases makes any difference, but I do it later anyway. Because of the posture of the baby, 90 percent of the residual mucus comes out. Suction doesn't usually get this much, although in some situations, suction continues to be important. We have done two hundred baths in the last few months. The father bathes the baby in the delivery room. Even with C-section, the husband bathes and massages the baby."

Here is Dr. Kliot's enthusiastic assessment of the method: "It is a gratifying delivery for the obstetrician, but family bonding is the strongest gain. Separation of the mother and baby can lead to rejection, and child abuse can be correlated with separation. I have been an obstetrician for years, but I never really saw the fascination of a baby before I used the Leboyer method."

"Babies love the Leboyer bath," says Dr. David Kliot, an obstetrician at the Brookdale Hospital Center. "But we have stayed with Leboyer's techniques because we feel they make childbirth safe." (Dr. David Kliot/Brookdale Hospital Medical Center)

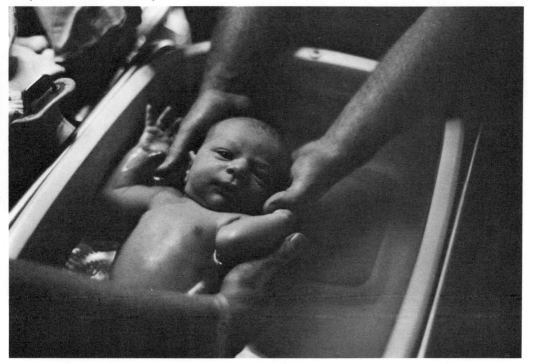

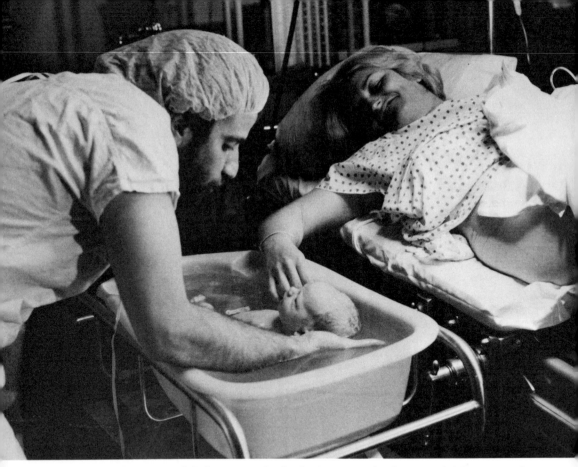

Parents and baby enjoy the bath. (Dr. David Kliot/Brookdale Hospital Medical Center)

A mother who delivered at a childbearing center said, "I don't know if I had a Leboyer birth or not. We brought a tape of our favorite songs, the only light was at the foot of the bed. Everything was sweet and soft. Everybody cared about everybody else's feelings and the baby didn't cry at all. Is that Leboyer?" Yes.

To Find a Leboyer Doctor: Your ICEA state coordinator (see Appendix I) will help you get in touch with a doctor who uses the Leboyer method. In the New York area, the Maternity Center Association, 48 East 92nd Street, tel.: 212–369–7300, will refer you to one.

THE NEED FOR A NEW MODEL

Not all big hospitals are hidebound. Old delivery rules are breaking down fast because institutions fear their obstetric patients will go elsewhere or have their babies at home.

Facing reality, five medical organizations, at this writing, are putting finishing touches on a joint statement endorsing sweeping changes in hospital obstetrics programs. The organizations are the American College of Obstetricians and Gynecologists, the American Academy of Pediatrics, the American College of Nurse-Midwives, the American Nurses' Association, and the Nurses Association of the American College of Obstetricians and Gynecologists. The provisions include:

1. Hospital-sponsored childbirth preparation classes for both parents.
2. Homelike "birthing rooms" for labor and delivery.
3. Permission for fathers to accompany women into delivery rooms and assist in births.
4. Permission for parents and babies to stay together during recovery.
4. No restrictions on other children's visits to their mother and new baby.

It's hard to say how long it will take hospitals to embrace these new concepts. Some already have. The following description of the innovative Hennepin County Medical Center in Minneapolis, Minnesota, can serve as an inspiration to activists for family-centered childbirth.

Since the new service started local women have been coming to Hennepin County Medical Center for childbirth in increasing numbers. They are referred by the hospital's clinic, health department clinics, other community clinics, and their friends and neighbors.

First, they are seen by a nurse-midwife, then by a doctor with the midwife. He decides, on the basis of her history and physical condition, if the patient can be part of the nurse-midwife program. Women with medical or obstetrical problems are referred to the physicians' clinic, but the midwife continues to participate in their care.

When she comes to the hospital for delivery, the woman is admitted directly to the room where she will stay throughout her hospitalization. She is seen and evaluated by both a midwife and an obstetric resident. If everything remains normal, she will labor, give birth, and remain afterward in the same room, keeping the baby with her. She may have all the people she wants present at the birth, including her other children. However, if young children are present, an adult must be with them to give constant supervision and care.

The regular cost is $800 for prenatal care, labor, birth, and the mother's and baby's stay at the hospital. Any special services such as cesarean section or newborn intensive care are extra. Most women stay three days, but exceptions can be made for earlier discharge, or the mother and baby may stay longer if there are problems. If the family goes home before the third day, the nurse-midwife visits daily through the third day, or the baby is brought back to the pediatric clinic.

If complications occur during pregnancy, labor, or birth, decisions for care are made by the physician. He delivers all breech, forceps, C-section, and twin births. All rooms have oxygen and suction equipment, with other equipment and supplies brought in on a portable cart at birth time.

No stirrups, arm restraints, or steel bar handles are used. Mothers take the baby immediately at birth, hold him as long as they wish, and may begin breast-feeding immediately. The temperature of the baby is maintained by wrapping him in blankets and keeping the room comfortably warm.

The father may and often does stay with the mother and baby all night. Care is individualized, and "routines" such as prepping, enema, and episiotomy are omitted unless found to be necessary.

Since the midwife service started, nurse-midwives have been delivering about one-quarter of the babies born at the hospital, and the total number of births at the hospital has increased by 17 percent, without any advertising or promotion. The administration is finding that these family-centered innovations are good business as well as good medicine!

The Childbearing Center: A "Homelike Delivery"

At their townhouse at 48 East 92 Street, New York, the Maternity Center Association is providing safe, satisfying, low-cost maternity care *outside* a hospital. Since the Childbearing Center began two years ago, eight centers modeled after it have opened around the country, and others are in the planning stage. After visiting the center, I believe that it may provide the best solution to many of the childbirth problems that beset us.

Babies in carefully screened low-risk situations are delivered by nurse-midwives (obstetrical backup is available), and then are discharged with their mothers just twelve hours later! The total cost of $575 includes extensive preparation for childbirth and child care, the delivery itself, and close supervision postpartum. This is about one-third what it costs to have a baby in most American hospitals, and one-fourth to one-fifth what it costs in New York City. Blue Cross and Blue Shield are participating in the program, and most participants have some coverage.

Everything is done to help families feel at home at the Childbearing Center. Women make relaxed visits throughout their pregnancy for classes, for careful examinations by obstetricians who are very alert to potential problems and screen them out, and for socialization with the friendly staff. Child care for older children is provided during these visits.

The deliveries themselves take place in a delightfully decorated three-room apartment with a terrace. Early labor is in the "living room," with midwives chatting, comforting, and fixing lunch and coffee for the parents. There are showers for the parents to use. Later the mother retires to the "bedroom" to give birth. The baby is born on a bed, in quiet and restful surroundings, with dim lights to protect his sensitive eyes (There is a spotlight at the foot of the bed.) Parents stay together all the time. After a few hours, the baby is seen by the pediatrician, and then the family goes home together. Older children are welcome to visit the mother and new baby whenever she feels ready to see them.

"Every delivery is a Leboyer delivery in principal," says nurse-midwife Betty Hosford. "The room is dim, there are soft voices, sometimes a warm bath for the baby." She adds proudly, "Our babies frequently come out crying, active, and pink. They are often superior to the official ten-point APGAR score. (This test is widely used in newborn examinations. It was developed by the late Dr. Virginia Apgar, and rates the newborn baby by observation of color, muscle tone, pulse reflex, irritability, and respiration. Usually it is given at one minute, five minutes and thirty minutes after birth.) The child-bearing center's babies often gain one-half pound over their birth weight in seven days, and the mother's milk supply usually comes in in twenty-four hours.

The director of the program is Ruth Lubic, a knowledgeable educator and a friendly, informal woman who has worked as a nurse-midwife. She says, "We're trying to provide the warm, personalized, human kind of service families say is missing from a hospital. We're particularly concerned that the mother and father not be separated from the baby."

"Homelike deliveries" are, for some people, much more satisfactory than home births. They provide medical safeguards, such as oxygen for the baby and an intravenous setup for the mother, that usually are not available at home, and a cooperating hospital is only eleven minutes away by car. An experienced staff is fully available before, during, and after delivery to support and reassure the parents. "We try to combine the best of two worlds," says Betty Hosford. "We are homelike with safety features."

When the program started, some doctors, such as Raymond Vande Weile from Columbia University's College of Physicians and Surgeons, thought that "an eleven-minute trip to the hospital is too much. The first five minutes are crucial." Others, like Dr. Alvin Donnenfeld, one of the obstetricians on call for the midwives, disagreed. "An ambulance covers all emergencies, and I don't think eleven minutes poses any greater risk."

Some women have had to be transported to the hospital during labor, yet the Childbearing Center has maintained a record of perfect safety and good outcome for both mother and child. "You can predict which situations are going bad with monitoring and scalp sampling," explains obstetrician Eugene Klochkoff of New York, who was associated with the program when it started.

There still is a good deal of controversy about whether the Childbearing Center is safe enough, and resistance to the project, even harassment, continues. Happily, so does the service.

The Office Birth Center

A number of obstetricians have told me, off the record, that many doctors have had the occasional experience of delivering a baby in the office because a patient absolutely refused to go to the hospital. Now a few doctors are equipping their offices as birth centers and recruiting registered nurses specially trained in obstetrics to help them. They're finding that they hardly can keep up with the demand for their services!

One such office birth center in Culver City, California, is called NACHIS (a Yiddish word meaning happiness) by its founder, Dr. Victor Berman. Until a few years ago, Dr. Berman did his "baby catching" in the Bradley tradition in hospitals. Then he and his wife Salee, a nurse practitioner qualified to counsel and examine pregnant patients and assist in their deliveries, decided to bring some NACHIS to their community.

Some three hundred births later, they have a perfect safety record.

"We have never had to hospitalize a mother, and we have never had to hospitalize a baby who has been delivered in the birth center," reports Dr. Berman. Problems have arisen, but they have been treated in the office with oxygen, suctioning equipment, drugs, IV fluid, and iron by

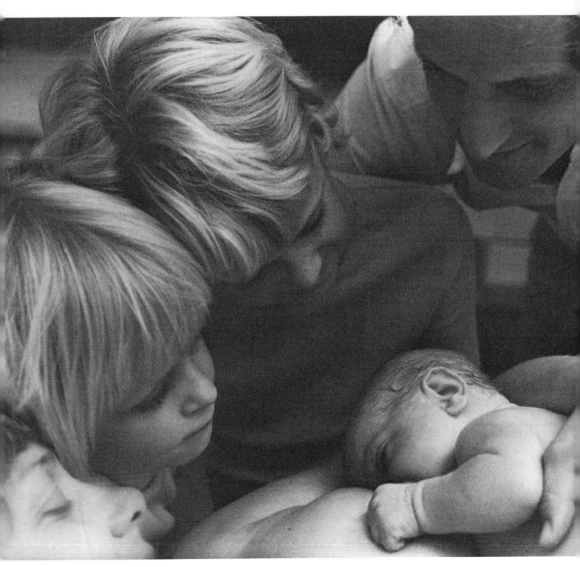

At the Nachis birth center in California the Harrison family gets to know Siri, who is only three minutes old in this photograph. (From the film: Alternative Childbirth, *Jay Hathaway Productions, courtesy American Academy of Husband-Coached Childbirth)*

mouth. "Just in case," the office is located only three minutes from a hospital.

Some of the people who come live hours away. Most stay only a few hours after birth, when the mother and baby are examined and discharged. As with all sound alternative settings, there is twenty-four-hour-a-day telephone support, and consultation and pediatric follow-up at home are available.

The service is not inexpensive—$1250 for office visits, delivery, and the use of the birth center—but it is less expensive than staying in a hospital and the office fee is covered by most patients' insurance. The parents who elect to come seem particularly well suited for this alternative setting. The women are confident of their bodies in a natural birth. They and their husbands are Bradley trained, united as a couple, and very enthusiastic. The doctor is a warm, ebullient, sensitive "father figure" in whom they feel trust and confidence. Even the climate is on their side. NACHIS is radiating out there in Culver City.

OUT-OF-HOSPITAL ALTERNATIVES

For referral to alternative settings and practitioners in your area:
Write or call NAPSAC, Marble Hill, Missouri 63764.
For most people, "alternative" has meant home birth. But there are other childbirth settings, with doctors or nurse-midwives as birth assistants, that are being developed to answer the public demand for safe, inexpensive, unregimented natural childbirth.

Eighty percent of the world's babies are delivered at home. While we have no exact figures, estimates are that almost 99 percent of American babies are born in hospitals. By contrast, in both modern industrial and developing nations, there are well-established home-birth midwifery programs, and fourteen of these nations have a lower infant mortality rate than we have!

The American perception of home birth is that it is intrinsically dangerous and old-fashioned, but there is a growing trend to home birth, particularly in the Far West. In other sections of the country, qualified assistance for home birth still is very hard to find and public prejudice against it is widespread. The major objection is that home birth is more dangerous for mother and baby. What are the facts?

Home Births: More Dangerous Than Hospital Deliveries?

Controversy rages on this question, with conflicting statistics supporting the views on either side. According to the American College of Obstetricians and Gynecologists (ACOG), *no* alternative to hospital birth is safe, even for normal childbirth. Their most recent official statement says, in part, "Labor and delivery, while a physiologic process, clearly present potential hazards to mother and fetus before and after birth. These hazards require standards of safety which are provided by the hospital setting and cannot be matched in the home setting."

The National Association of Parents and Professionals for Safe Alternatives in Childbirth (NAPSAC), has an opposing view. It maintains that home births, properly arranged, are as safe or safer than hospital deliveries, and "if at the present time home births do present an additional risk, no small part of that risk would be due to willful negligence by a hostile medical establishment that, by refusing prenatal care and hospital backup, seems to be attempting to make home births as hazardous as possible in order to make their hospitals appear safer."

ACOG buttresses its views with these statistics: While hospital births have gone way up in the last twenty-five years, maternal mortality has almost disappeared and infant mortality has been halved. The safest, lowest-risk situation can suddenly escalate into an emergency—for example, a sudden hemorrhage needing massive transfusion. At a NAPSAC convention, Dr. Richard Aubry of ACOG said, "One of the reasons the low-risk patient does so well is *because* of the hospital." He also presented alarming statistics from Oregon that show that the mortality rate for home-birth babies is twice that for hospital-born babies. (A recent Hawaiian study also indicates that more home babies die, as does a third statistic from Maine. In Hawaii, the death rate for home babies was three times that of hospital-born ones.)

Home-birth advocates disavow these statistics. They point to the long history of safe deliveries by the Frontier Nursing Service, whose nurse-midwives have delivered thousands of babies in poor homes since 1925 with maternal and infant mortality rates consistently lower than the national average. This same excellent outcome was consistently reported in The Chicago Homebirth Service, where young doctors in training delivered thousands of babies into slum homes with a better outcome than that for the same population in Chicago hospitals at the same time.

NAPSAC explains the alarming new statistics this way: "Most home births today are not being reported. The ones that have complications, problems, or fatalities. . . . A recent California study revealed that only 25 percent of home-birth couples registered their babies. . . . One reason is that they are upbraided and questioned rudely by the authorities." And NAPSAC's research director, Dr. Lewis Mehl of California, recently completed a study of a matched sample of two thousand babies, half born in the hospital and half at home, delivered by the same doctors. "The only difference was that hospital-born babies had a harder time. . . . Death rates were essentially the same."

The reason for this conflicting evidence seems clear to me. If you want a home birth that is as safe as a hospital birth, or safer, get a qualified assistant to help you deliver. Frontier Nursing Service has qualified nurse-midwives. Chicago Homebirth used doctors in training and supervised them closely. In Dr. Mehl's recent studies, home-birth assistants were trained doctors. How many of the couples in the Oregon, Hawaii, and Maine statistics had qualified help at home?

It also is vital to arrange the home properly, to make backup arrangements for medical attention and hospitalization in case of emergency, and to be sure throughout your pregnancy that you remain "low risk." If any of these safeguards is *not* possible, I recommend that couples extend themselves, traveling a distance if necessary, to find a family-centered facility. It's the support of the surroundings, not the decor, that matters.

Who Is Having Home Birth

Psychotherapist and childbirth educator Lester Hazell studied some of the people in California who are giving birth at home today, and her findings shed some interesting light on their life-styles and motivations. Despite the common belief that most home-birth families are "counterculture," in her study 90 percent were middle class, lived in single-family dwellings, owned cars and televisions, were gainfully employed, and had some college education. They had decided on home birth out of conviction, not monetary need, ignorance, or rebellion against society. In other words, very few were hippies, but many were dissatisfied hospital consumers.

Here are some of the reasons they opted for home birth:
1. I wanted a relaxed environment.
2. I didn't want unfamiliar and unsupportive attendants.
3. I preferred to be attended by supportive women attendants.
4. I wanted to avoid excessive intervention.
5. I didn't want aggressive obstetrical intervention—rupturing of membranes, routine induction, elective cesarean in breech, etc.
6. I didn't want a routine episiotomy.
7. I wanted to labor and deliver in the same place.
8. I wanted to avoid separation of family members after birth.
9. I wanted to avoid being separated from a sick baby after birth.
10. I wanted to breast-feed immediately and on demand.
11. I wanted to avoid a long hospital stay.
12. I didn't want routine "prepping."
13. I preferred to move around during labor, and to eat and drink.
14. I wanted to choose my birth assistant.

Midwife Nancy Mills, in her presentation to NAPSAC, talked about the very different group of people she has worked with. "A very high percentage of these women have no prenatal care at all. . . . In the area we're in, the nearest obstetrical care is up to two hours' drive. The women were just not coming in."

In the clinic where she works now, she noted, "I am continually called by members of several churches in the area." The growth of yogic childbirth also indicates that home birth sometimes is being selected for spiritual reasons.

Mills's population commonly expressed these reasons:

1. I prefer a midwife and a home delivery.
2. There was no doctor available.
3. I didn't like the hospital.
4. I didn't want to leave my children and family.
5. I prefer to have a woman with me.
6. I can't afford a hospital.

SOME LOCAL DOCTORS AND MOTHERS TALK
ABOUT HOME BIRTH TODAY

To get some unofficial responses about home birth from doctors, I asked some for their opinions "off the record."

First, those who used to do home births but don't do them anymore

"Liability is a serious problem. You can't insulate yourself against it Possibly, home deliveries are less sound than they used to be."

The intimacy of a home birth cannot be matched in any other setting. (Courtesy John and Barbara Barosa)

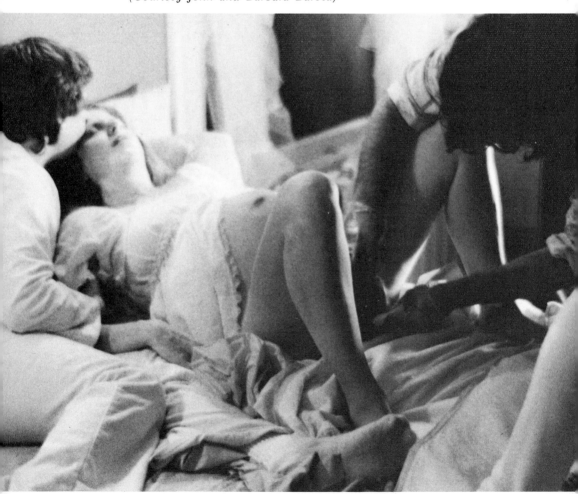

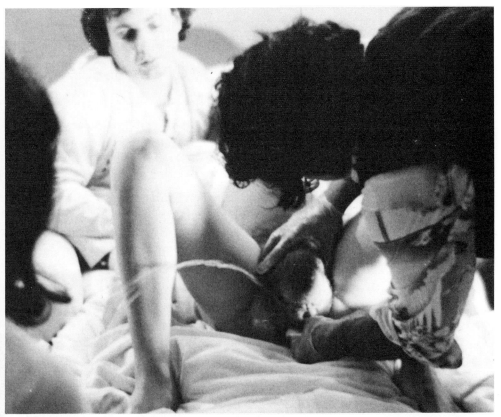

The normal breaking of the waters signals that the baby will be coming soon. (Courtesy John and Barbara Barosa)

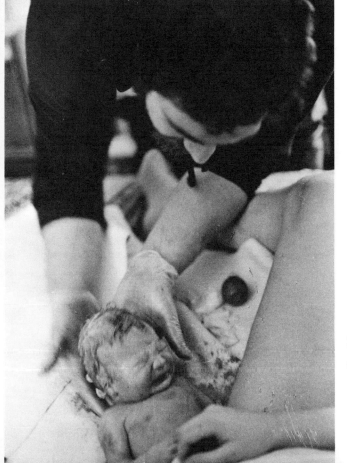

In many home births the "prepared" father can be "baby catcher." (John Crockett)

"The patients loved them. In those days, there was a good backup system. You could do an operation for cesarean section right there on the kitchen table, but there is no backup now. They're just not practical."

There still are a few doctors around who will deliver babies at home and say so publicly. It is their conviction that the woman has the right of free choice, and they are dedicated to natural childbirth.

Other doctors prefer not to be so open about their willingness to participate in home birth, partly because of the official position of their medical association and partly because they don't want to be flooded with requests they can't handle. One of them told me, "I try to convince the patient to go to the hospital, and I also try to make the hospital more flexible. But if the hospital doesn't give the patient any choice, it, as well as the mother, must take responsibility if anything goes wrong."

Another simply stated his philosophy: "I think a home delivery is a warm and wonderful emotional experience, though it has certain risks. I will take the risks if the mother does."

Most couples I spoke to were truly enthusiastic about their experience: "My husband was on one side of me and Peter [her little boy] was on the other. I was supported by their love. I believe childbirth should be a family experience."

Another describes how nicely things worked out: "The baby came about five o'clock in the morning. We have an upstairs and a downstairs, and my little girl slept all the way through. When she got up at seven and came downstairs, we said, 'You have a little sister.' My next-door neighbor scrambled some eggs, and we all had breakfast together—the doctor, the family, and my friend. I felt well enough to walk slowly up the stairs afterward, my husband carried the baby, and I took a rest in my own bed."

But other women who have had home births with good physical outcomes feel they missed the emotional support of a hospital delivery. These women and their husbands felt too alone, too overwhelmed by the responsibility, because they had no family or friends to support them.

Here is one such report: "Everything went fine, but to tell the truth, my husband and I were scared and lonely. We have no family and had to handle everything ourselves before the doctor came. No one was there

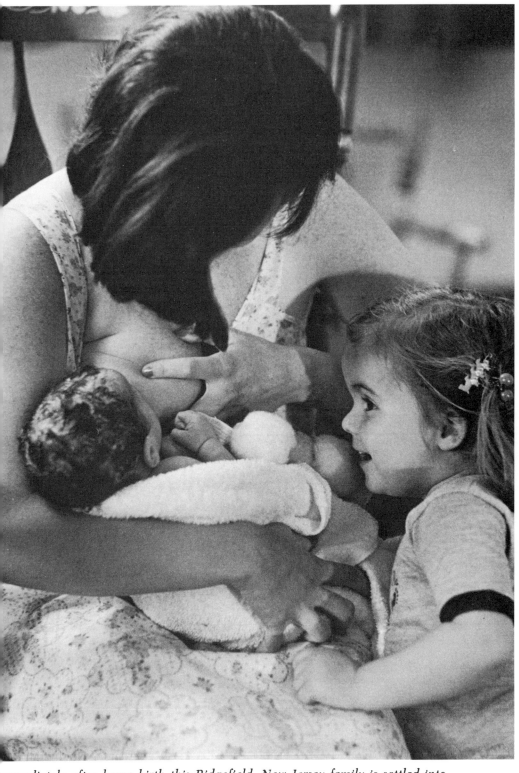

mmediately after home birth this Ridgefield, New Jersey family is settled into ts new routine. (Alison Ehrlich Wachstein, from Pregnant Moments, Morgan *Morgan, 1978)* afterward, except the doctor, who came to check the baby every day. We decided that for the next baby I would go to the hospital. The doctor, the same man who delivered me at home, was able to get the hospital to do things my way. I had a private room, and I went home as soon as I felt well enough. I only stayed overnight and part of the next day, but while I was there, I had the feeling that everyone was working to help me. For us, it was a much easier experience."

Everyone agrees that the mother's health, the course of the pregnancy, and good home circumstances are equally important. "Good sense is the most important factor," said one doctor. "When a couple is sure that this is what they want, then it's up to them to find qualified help."

Getting Help with Home Birth

As you can see by the lengthy referral list at the end of this section, it is *not* impossible to find a qualified expert and the education you need to prepare properly for home birth today. In addition to those sources, your own obstetrician and local childbirth educator may know of a qualified local person who will help you. The two parent support groups on the list are mushrooming in size. The Association for Childbirth at Home, Inc. (ACHI), which started in 1972, already has 250 leaders, trainers, and groups in the United States, Canada, and England. It expects to double in size this year. Home-Oriented Maternity Experience (HOME), whose monthly meetings are patterned on the La Leche League method of mutual support, had 35 groups at this writing, with 150 leader applicants waiting to be trained. Of the two, HOME has the larger list of qualified assistants to whom you will be referred.

Both these groups also provide excellent education for home birth, particularly ACHI, which offers an intensive twenty-four-hour course, a comprehensive manual, and a great deal of information about nutrition, home preparation, obstetrics, and aftercare of the mother and baby. They teach you how to make backup arrangements and how to choose a qualified assistant. HOME also has a guide, in which the advantages of home birth are discussed, along with responsibilities, equipment, birth procedures, psychological aspects, medical considerations, breast-feeding, nutrition, and parenting. If you are planning a home birth and can afford the ACHI course, begin there. Then join the free HOME support group in your neighborhood until the birth.

Both groups provide an important service. Unfortunately, some of the people who go to them for help get so enthusiastic about the information that they think they are qualified to deliver the baby themselves.

I checked with Doris Haire about the danger of cord entanglement (it occurs in one-fourth to one-third of deliveries) in home birth. She assured me that, "the cord around the neck has not been shown to produce any adverse effects if the membranes are intact. The amniotic fluid is a cushion that prevents strong uterine muscles from compressing the umbilical cord against the fetus's head or body. In the majority of cases, membranes do not rupture until labor is advanced or the baby is actually being born."

Still, too many things can happen that unqualified family and friends aren't prepared to deal with calmly. Home birth *can* be safe, and fathers often can have the thrill of delivering their babies themselves. But they should do so under the careful, experienced eye of an expert!

If you do decide to give birth at home, prepare properly with all the necessary equipment outlined in the ACHI and HOME manuals, and make good arrangements for both you and your baby to have privacy, rest, and care afterward. Another adult will be needed to take over the home responsibilities and to provide care for you and the baby. A pediatrician or visiting nurse should come in each day to check the baby. In the excitement, don't forget to register the baby and get a birth certificate!

Important Guidelines for Safe Home Birth

1. Get excellent prepartum care. Be sure you are completely "low risk" by your confinement date.
2. Get excellent education for home birth. Take the ACHI course, which prepares your partner to assist and educates you both to know in detail what to expect in normal childbirth. Join a HOME parent group for support during pregnancy.
3. Get an expert assistant, well experienced with home birth. Both parent organizations advise you how to select one.
4. Prepare your home with proper equipment.
5. Arrange for pediatric follow-up in advance.
6. Arrange in advance for emergency hospitalization and transportation to the hospital.

7. Arrange for constant help at home to care for you and the baby, at least for three days and preferably for a week or longer.

These guidelines provide only a bare outline of what really is necessary to make home birth work for you. Both parents need the emotional support of friends and family before, during, and after birth. In addition, they need to work out the fears and dependencies that interfere with responsible and comfortable functioning. The program described below is a unique attempt to provide the professional team service, emotional support, and practical assistance needed for home birth.

A Model Home Birth Program

In July 1977, NAPSAC research director and family doctor Lewis Mehl, social worker Gail Peterson, a nurse-midwife, and a nurse-practitioner all joined as a team practice and opened the doors of the Berkeley Family Health Center, which is providing a model program NAPSAC hopes will be used by others in years to come.

An intrinsic part of their practice is extensive research to determine the psychological and social factors that create hazards in home birth; psycho-physiological factors in the pathology of childbirth, such as uterine inertia; and factors that cause postpartum depression. "Because people want home births, we need this information to screen for risk. We also are counseling to improve their situation. We are trying to provide a total psychological and physical approach," says Dr. Mehl.

Although you needn't be pregnant to go to the Berkeley Health Center, most clients are. First, they see a nurse practitioner or the doctor to find out about the service, and then Ms. Peterson sees them for a social work screening to find out what they will need in terms of education and information and also to assess their needs for help during pregnancy with personality, marital, or social factors. By the time their initial contact with her is complete, couples have begun planning for their childbirth.

There are a number of important options all the way through. Couples can select either home or hospital delivery. They can be part of a prenatal group or be seen alone for prenatal care. Most people choose to be in a group of four couples, which gives them the opportunity to give and get peer, as well as professional, support.

Preparation for labor classes are realistic and imaginative; slides and audio tapes of labor are used for psychological preparation, for example. Individual counseling services are available throughout, and couples can continue in their original groups for "well-baby" care. At the Berkeley Family Health Center, this means routine examinations plus infant developmental information, including suggestions for interventions to assure optimal development. There is also a monthly open house to give couples additional opportunities to make friends, compare news, and get support.

Home birth is carefully planned. People are encouraged to have three or four persons present during birth in case extra help is needed, and afterward to take care of the home and the mother and baby. Although thus far it hasn't been necessary to hospitalize a mother, provisions are always made for admitting a woman to the obstetrical service in the hospital closest to her home in case of emergency.

After birth, there are three home visits by members of the team, office visits of mother and baby at seven days and four weeks, and postpartum classes, often with the original four-couple prepartum group. The fee for the entire service is approximately $600.

A unique feature of the center is that it provides care for the entire family, not just the pregnant mother and newborn baby, and all the professionals work together as a team. Dr. Mehl says, "I am very pro-family doctor. I feel it improves care to have the same physician working across several generations. That way, he can appreciate the whole kin system— how the parents' psychological and physical problems affect the children, and vice versa."

This seamless service supports people from one life stage to the next. Most Americans don't have sufficient family and community support, and it is unlikely this will change in contemporary society. Berkeley Health Center is an updated family practice that provides psychological as well as medical expertise, and the opportunity to form friendships with other young families. Set up specifically to make home birth safer and more successful, it also is providing an excellent model for the family practice of the future.

Dr. Mehl and his co-workers welcome inquiries from other professionals who are interested in starting similar services. Both clients and professionals can reach them at 2522 Dana Street, Suite 201, Berkeley, California 94702.

HOME-BIRTH REFERRALS

For referral to a qualified birth attendant: Write to:

1. Home-Oriented Maternity Experience (HOME), 511 York Avenue, Takoma Park, Washington, D. C. 20012. Referral is free. There are local support groups (voluntary membership fee) and a low-cost preparatory manual. This organization has the largest list of obstetricians, nurse-midwives, and lay midwives.

2. The Association for Childbirth at Home, Inc. (ACHI), Box 1219, Cerritos, California 90701. Referral is free. There is a thorough training program, including a training manual, for couples planning home birth. The cost is $60–$75 for six classes.

3. The American College of Home Obstetrics, 664 North Michigan, Suite 600, Chicago, Illinois 60611. Referral is free. This is a fairly young organization that started in the Chicago area and has spread to other parts of the country. It has a small list of obstetricians and family practitioners who are willing to go on record as attending home births.

4. The National Midwife Association, P.O. Box 163, Princeton, New Jersey 08540. Another young organization of lay midwives who are working to establish standards of practice. The association will refer you to a qualified member, free.

5. Call the local medical center that has a nurse-midwife unit. The nurse-midwives there will refer you to a private practitioner in your area.

12

Step 4
Selecting the Best Pediatrician

You have only one more expert to find before the baby comes. I suggest you meet a number of pediatricians *now*—while you have the time, are still independent, and your critical faculties are clearest.

In some advanced practices, like the university-connected Ambulatory Pediatric Service directed by Dr. Catherine De Angelis in Madison, Wisconsin, women are encouraged to come in early in pregnancy. "We meet the patient immediately after conception," the doctor says. In most communities, however, pediatricians aren't part of childbirth teams, so if you want to meet yours before the baby comes, you'll have to make your own appointment. Doctors assure me they would be delighted to meet prospective patients any time.

Most doctors work on their own or in a small group, with a nurse to help them, but a few forward-looking pediatricians are adding to their staffs to get mothers started in an optimal way. One group practice, in La Jolla, California, has added a "professional grandmother." She visits mothers in the hospital after birth, and then once again at home, to answer questions about feeding and bathing the infant. (Grandmothers today will remember that this is exactly the service that was offered to them, free of charge, by the local Visiting Nurse Association.)

Another group of pediatricians, in Long Island, New York, is very interested in helping breast-feeding mothers. They have hired three nurses who are experienced breast-feeders. Each is assigned to a group of mothers. All are available during the day, and some evenings, for office and telephone consultations.

You may not be fortunate enough to live near such an advanced practice, but you will be able to get good personal recommendations from your childbirth teacher, classmates, and obstetrician. If your obstetrician promotes breast-feeding, he's very likely to know the two or three best pediatric practices that can help you.

If you want to be discharged early from the hospital, you'll need a pediatrician who will agree to see you and the baby at home or in his office the first few days. While all the pediatricians I called at random assured me they would be willing to take on this responsibility, some had more enthusiasm for and familiarity with the practice than others.

After the baby comes, you will find that the support of a trustworthy, easily accessible pediatrician is worth its weight in gold. Yet a pediatrician you can relate to in a relaxed and personal way, whose philosophy on child rearing is close to your own, often is hard to find. Most pediatricians are friendly, cheerful people, but they tend to be extremely busy, even more so than other doctors.

It is not unusual for a pediatrician to be hard to reach on the telephone except during the "telephone hour," 7 A.M. to 8 A.M., when you are likely to get a frustrating busy signal. Some doctors have nurses who can screen their calls during the day and will respond immediately when they feel it's important, but others actually take the telephone off the hook while they're examining patients.

I believe the personality of the doctor is reflected in the way he manages his practice. Some seem able to work in an organized, even easygoing way. With others, you will find yourself getting exhausted in the waiting room and distracting your fretful baby until it is his turn to be examined. Some doctors do keep to appointment times, take plenty of time to talk, come to your home at the hour you expect them, and communicate respect and concern for the mother as an individual. Unlike a good restaurant, the quality of a doctor should not be gauged by the number of people crowding the waiting area. A quiet waiting room simply reflects a different style of practice, just as differences in play facilities may reflect the doctor's responsiveness to the temperament of waiting youngsters.

Costs of pediatric service vary considerably also. Fees generally have gone up a lot in the last few years, reflecting the rise in malpractice insurance and other expenses with which doctors have to cope. Among the doctors I interviewed, office visits ranged between $10 and $15 (with shots extra), and $15 to $25 was common for home visits. "Annual contracts" have been discarded. Insurance coverage, for most people, is minimal. GHI pays $5 for an office visit, $8 for a home visit. Only the most expensive Blue Cross policy covers routine pediatric visits, and the reimbursement is small. In some areas, there are private insurance plans (such as HIP) that cover the whole family's medical needs, including obstetric and pediatric care. Many are prohibitively expensive, but coverage may be a job benefit. You will be visiting the pediatrician's office once a month at first (if everything goes smoothly), and then once every six weeks during the baby's first year.

If you drive a car, it isn't necessary to use the services of the doctor closest to home. Most people want a doctor whose office is accessible in bad weather, but it's worthwhile making a longer trip if there are special needs.

For older female children, you might consider going to a female pediatrician, with whom your girls will feel more at ease during vaginal and breast examinations. They also provide an excellent role model. In the early years, however, the doctor's personality and ability to relate well to children is far more important than sex.

You'll be making many important decisions the first year, particularly about how often and what to feed the baby, so it's important to thoroughly check your doctor's attitudes and philosophy about infant feeding.

Is weight gain very important to him? Doctors differ about what is a healthy weight gain, and recent findings that fat babies become fat adults are changing the views of many. How does your pediatrician feel about solid supplements? Here doctors differ a great deal. I recommend the conservative approach—avoiding solids altogether in the first months—as healthiest for the new baby.

If you're breast-feeding, your baby will seem hungry most of the time in the first months. You'll need some practical help in determining how long each feeding should last, which will depend on the condition of your nipples. A doctor's attitude toward breast-feeding also is reflected in his practice. Many doctors I spoke to still do not refer mothers to La Leche League. Others strongly support breast-feeding in a practical manner by hiring experienced breast-feeding nurses to help inexperienced mothers with day-to-day support and problem solving. It's a good idea if you're breast-feeding to keep on your side table a good how-to book such as Karen Pryer's *Nursing Your Baby* (New York, Pocket Books) or the *La Leche Manual* (or others on the La Leche list, which can be ordered from them).

If your doctor tends to be anxious about weight gain, he'll probably recommend pureed banana and applesauce within weeks to guarantee it. Allergists are discovering a remarkable number of teenagers with banana allergy today, so this practice cannot be recommended routinely. If you're breast-feeding, the doctor may suggest solids instead of milk supplements, but a formula is better for the baby's digestion, if not for encouraging breast-feeding. However, some women are finding that it's possible to use breast and bottle interchangeably (see chapter 8).

If you find it difficult to maintain a good communication with the pediatrician when special problems arise, it's neither unethical nor unwise to consult another doctor. Your responsibility for staying in charge does not end when you make your first selection of a pediatrician. Doctors differ in their medical management of some conditions, like allergies and celiac disease. They differ about how and when to use antibiotics. If your baby is having problems that do not seem to be getting better, it makes perfect sense to change to another doctor in whose expertise you have more confidence. There are subspecialties in pediatrics, as in all branches of medicine, and your own pediatrician can recommend a good specialist for any special problem your baby may be having.

Keep in mind that mothers and babies are so tuned in to each other in the early months that a fretful infant may be responding to nothing more than a mother's anxiety and depression. If this is so, psychological help for the mother and family couseling to help a couple make supportive changes in household management may be the best answer.

Once you have established good working relationships with the experts you need and have made good arrangements for delivery, you can relax and enjoy the rest of your pregnancy with a clear mind.

In Part Four, I will talk about good household arrangements, finding friends, and locating special resources in your community to help you and your husband move into parenting with more assurance and pleasure.

Part Four:

AFTER THE BABY COMES

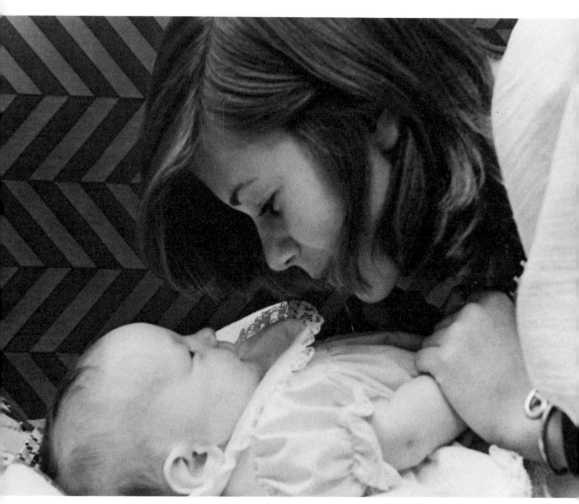

The two of us—a special feeling. (From the Parenting Pictures film: The Cesarean Birth Experience, *Courter Films and Associates)*

13

Adjusting to Parenthood

The most important—and ignored—part of the childbirth experience is portpartum. After the baby comes, the changes in your life will be tremendous, and you will need as much support and help from other people as you can get. Here are some of the reasons why.

Somehow, most people never are emotionally ready for a first baby. The required reordering of priorities is just too enormous to conceive of in advance. After living your whole life as an individual, caring first for yourself, it is impossible to imagine what it feels like to have to put someone else first all the time. You and your husband will not be in charge of your own lives and your own time again, until the children are grown and gone!

The ability to sleep soundly often is the first sacrifice. Every little noise awakens the new mother, even if she always slept undisturbed before. Every breath the baby draws is magnified through the megaphone of her anxiety. New parents cannot eat a meal without feeling concerned that the baby might cry. They can't go to the bathroom and close the door, or go out together for an evening, without feelings of anxiety. They are always "on"—available, concerned, involved—and, too often, worried and anxious.

Years later, when the children are adolescents or young adults, parents recall those early years nostalgically. "It was easy then," they will tell you. "All we had to do was feed the baby, hold him, or change him. Little children, little troubles." What they forget is how it felt to be chronically tired in the first months, how their ears literally hurt after hours of strained listening for the baby's cries while they were trying to rest, sleep, read, or entertain.

The transition from a personal life to parenthood probably is the most difficult and demanding time of people's lives. If you have any doubt about it, ask a young couple as they celebrate their survival into the sec ond year of parenthood. Watch them exchange knowing, rueful glances. They won't say for sure it was all worth it, but they will admit how much they have changed. We human beings seem to need the tremendous challenge of becoming parents in order, finally, to grow up. The maturational process includes taking care of the new baby. It works, but it also hurts!

If you don't realize that pain is part of the process, you will blame yourself for finding everything so hard and wonder what is wrong with you. The best way to beat that kind of self put-down is to become acquainted with other new parents. When you have a chance to communicate candidly and compare notes among yourselves, you'll all feel much better.

New parenthood is particularly hard on mothers. Women today are used to being independent, free to come and go. With a baby, they feel isolated, stuck, bored, and claustrophobic. Even if they had looked forward to temporary retirement from their jobs, they find themselves envying their husbands as they leave for work in the morning: "At least he can get out of the house!"

In the early years, many women make the mistake of settling for superficial and competitive neighborhood socialization rather than forming friendships with compatible women who share their values in child rearing. Your husband may be your best friend, but you will find that the companionship of other women is very important, particularly when the children are small. Research reveals that while women bring their complaints and anxieties first to their doctors, and then to their husbands, it is from other women that they feel they get the best help.

New fathers are under considerable strain, too. Many are concerned about what is going on at home while they're working. Like their wives, they're fighting fatigue most of the time, worrying about how they will function during the day: "At lease she can take a nap," they will tell you enviously. In our inflationary and insecure times, young husbands worry about meeting expenses, about the future, about getting ahead. Many feel that nothing in their marriage is free and easy anymore—not sex, not having dinner together, not going for a car ride.

As Andrea Boroff Eagan of HealthRight, a national woman's health organization, notes, "The nuclear family really doesn't work at that time, unless both parents are free to be home all the time." This is the time of a couple's life when they would welcome the participation and help of

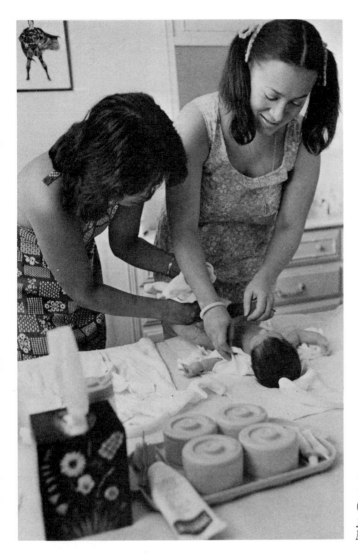

A sister or a friend can help develop confidence in the new mother at the beginning. (Alison Ehrlich Wachstein, from Pregnant Moments, Morgan & Morgan, 1978)

grandparents, brothers and sisters, and friends, but very often they don't get it. They feel hesitant to reach out to peers for what they feel they should be getting from their families, so they struggle alone through the early years of parenthood.

People with a growing family can always use help, support, and understanding. For many, the coming of each new baby is a tumultuous time, until the baby settles in, until the whole family readjusts to include him. How do you tell the first child about the new one coming? Should you go to the hospital or have a home birth to avoid separation from the other children? What is the best way to handle sibling jealousy? Once you're a parent, there always seems to be a new problem around the corner. Parenting is like a constant postgraduate education.

The first six weeks of the new lifetime curriculum are, in many ways, the most critical. Let's explore that period first.

THE FIRST SIX WEEKS

"People are isolated. They don't get enough sleep. No one quite realizes the responsibility of taking care of a new baby, particularly when they're not feeling well physically. The couple's relationship is under a strain. Lovemaking is off. All couples go through a crisis that lasts at least six weeks." This is the assessment of Elisabeth Bing, author, childbirth educator, and director of the Elisabeth Bing Center for Parents in New York.

Please understand that this state of affairs is not inevitable—just very common. Part of the reason, as I have said, is sociological. But there is another, equally important cause. Pregnant women simply don't absorb very much about what motherhood will be like, no matter how much their childbirth teachers and authors like me try to tell them. Instead, they hold on to all kinds of illusions, which are a lot more comforting than reality.

Once thrust into the new situation, the recuperating mother doesn't have either the psychic or physical resilience to cope serenely or with self-confidence. Little things, like finding a neighborhood teenager to watch the baby for an hour between feedings, become mountainous tasks. New mothers often are afraid to drive, to get the baby ready to go out, or to stay alone at home with the baby. They overreact, panic, blame themselves, question their feelings for the baby, wonder if they are suited for motherhood. Later on, they look back in wonderment at some of the things they thought about and did.

"A week after the baby came, I really flipped out. I said to my husband, 'I have a good idea. Your mother likes the baby. I don't. I'll give *her* the baby and I'll go to Europe.'" Outlandish thoughts like these are quite common and not "sick." Andrea Eagan explains, "It's a process. You're finishing out the reproductive process. How you feel in those first weeks is not the way you'll feel later. Most people, after three weeks, are complaining bitterly. But three weeks after that, they feel better."

In my experience, they will surely feel better if they do something about the things that are bothering them. If they're overtired, they need sleep. If they're claustrophobic, they need to get out of the house—without the baby. If they're isolated, they need to join a group to make friends. It has been found that when mothers begin postpartum classes in the first few weeks after the baby's birth, their emotional and physical recuperation is easier and more rapid. It's a very good idea to arrange to begin your postpartum classes *before* the baby comes. Chances are that paying for them in advance and promising that you will come will give you the incentive you need to get going.

Now, while you are pregnant, can you project yourself into the emotional state you're likely to be in the first six weeks after childbirth? It's difficult, but not impossible. Here are some exercises and suggestions I have found useful in preparing women for the emotional aftermath of childbirth:

Exercise 1. Remember back to when you first went away to college, or when you started to work at your first full-time job. Do you recall how scared and overwhelmed you felt? Most important, remember your feelings of regret and anger at yourself because you had willingly gotten yourself into that situation. Then remember how long it took to adjust, and finally to enjoy the new situation. It takes just about as long to enjoy new parenthood.

Exercise 2. Remember how you felt when you were learning to drive a car. Your arms and back muscles ached. Your neck was stiff, and your eyes burned. Most important, remember how you felt about yourself, how you thought you were impossibly clumsy and stupid, sure to have an accident and kill somebody. Everybody else seemed to be learning to drive effortlessly, while you thought you'd never learn. But you did, and now you're a pretty good driver.

Exercise 3. This is a real-life project, guaranteed to give you a taste of parenthood in advance. Get a puppy or a kitten during your pregnancy. It will need comforting in your bed. You'll find it jumping in your bed or at the doorknob, impatient to be walked at the crack of dawn. You'll have to be available to walk it and feed it. You'll need a pet-sitter to get away from home, even for a day. Whew, what a job! Little by little, you'll incorporate this new bundle of responsibility into your daily life.

By the time the new baby comes, your beloved pet will be great company. It will greet you when you come home from the hospital, and keep you and the baby company on rainy days. Why did it ever seem hard to take care of a new puppy? You certainly get back a lot more than you give.

Of course, taking care of a young pet is a lot less worrisome than taking care of a baby. It's just a taste of the responsibility, but the feelings are similar.

You will notice that each of these three exercises highlights a psychological problem. In the first, it was the feeling that you made a choice and now are stuck with it. In the second, it was lack of confidence that you would ever be able to acquire the necessary skills to manage the required task. The third exercise required you to deal with new and unexpected feelings—the concern and anxiety that come with responsibility for the survival of a helpless, living creature. If these three elements combine into obsessive ideas that torment you after the baby comes, you may work yourself into an agitated depression, called the "baby blues" or postpartum depression. Just what is this condition, and what can you do to avoid it?

POSTPARTUM DEPRESSION

Feelings of agitation and depression are so common after childbirth that some experts consider them inevitable. There is disagreement about whether the condition is triggered most by physical, psychological, or environmental causes. The central question is: Would anyone recuperating from childbirth get depressed under poor environmental conditions, or is postpartum depression simply a surfacing of a life-long problem of the mother?

Sheila Kitzinger, who estimates that about two-thirds of women suffer depression after childbirth, believes much postpartum depression is a kind of growing pain. She says, "There is no remedy, no miracle drug, for the suffering that is the necessary accompaniment of growing up."

On the other hand, traditional psychoanalysts think that postpartum depression is a pathological condition arising from the new mother's problem of separation—from both her own mother and the new baby who has left her body. Whether or not a woman gets depressed, they say, depends mostly on her upbringing and her relationship with her own mother.

A third view is that postpartum depression often is triggered by an emotionally upsetting birth experience, which interferes with the mother's normal ability to bond with her baby. That is the finding of Dr. Lewis Mehl and Gail Peterson, who concur with the observation of Dr. Helene Deutsch, a world-famous psychiatrist of the 1940s, who said that "obstetrical interference can change the experience of delivery to a disappointing one, dominated by horror, and this can prevent the mother from developing love for the newborn." Deutsch noted that the mother's passivity and lack of participation in the delivery could leave something unresolved in her. "She experiences the whole process uncreatively, not as giving life to a child, but as an operation that has removed something harmful, something she now must confront in the outside world."

No one is completely sure of the cause of postpartum blues, but current observations of mothers who do not bond normally and later reject their children is leading experts to believe that the normal bonding process is important in preventing postpartum depression. If the mother cannot feel love for her baby and experiences him as an alien, frightening person rather than as part of herself, the whole reason for her existence as a mother is brought into question. All the work, all the endless hours of caretaking, have no meaning or pleasure without love.

In my clinical experience as a psychotherapist, it is often the combination of a traumatic childbirth and a poor doctor-patient relationship that produces postpartum depression. Here is a typical example of a mother, previously stable and healthy, who plummeted into a postpartum depression almost immediately after childbirth, and stayed there, despite good hospital arrangements, support at home, and successful breast-feeding:

"I started to cry in the hospital and I'm still crying. I had a breech birth and the doctor tried to induce the baby. It didn't work and he said, 'Your baby is as stubborn as you are.' When he was doing internals during labor, he hurt me very badly, and I screamed at him to stop. He walked out of the room in a huff, and my husband had to run after him and beg him to come back. It was a mess all the way through. The baby's leg was twisted and my husband yelled, 'What has that doctor done to my baby?'

"The childbirth teacher came to see me in the hospital afterward. She said she had known I'd have a hard time because I didn't like the doctor. Why didn't she tell me that while I was pregnant so I could switch to someone else? I didn't know my feelings would matter so much during the delivery.

"Now I just feel sorry I have a baby. I hate my life. I feel guilty toward my husband, but I can't help it. Every time I remember what happened at the hospital, I cry. How did I get into this mess?"

Some mothers report that their problems stemmed from lack of sup-

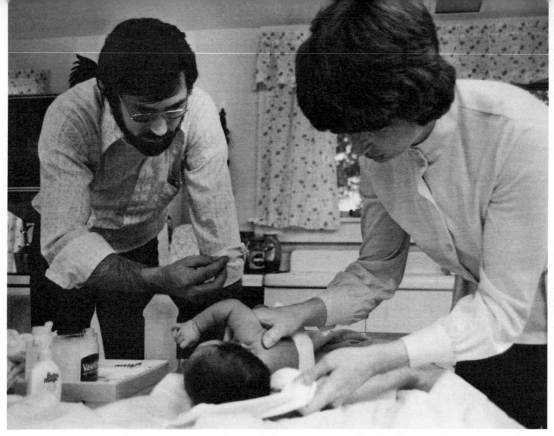

The best assistant in the world is a consistently helpful husband. (From the Parenting Pictures film: Are You Ready for the Postpartum Experience?, *Courter Films and Associates)*

port at home rather than what happened during the childbirth: "I had a beautiful birth experience. But I had breast-feeding problems and a difficult baby. The worst thing was not having anyone to turn to for advice or help." Another says, "It was the isolation with my baby after I came home from the hospital that was devastating. My husband went away on a two-week business trip, and when he came back, I was in such bad shape I had to be hospitalized. He was lucky we both were still alive."

Even though postpartum depression feels agonizing when you're going through it, it usually is not seriously pathological and actually represents a floundering effort to integrate and begin to function as a mother. The condition responds best, and fairly quickly, to consistent understanding, patience, and sympathy.

What helps women most is an emotionally supportive environment. Having helpful, loving people around can heal the wounds of a lifetime, as well as the recent traumas of a poor childbirth experience. Professional psychotherapists attempt to provide that loving support both in the office and by arranging for a better home situation.

Perhaps the professionel can listen more calmly than the family to the

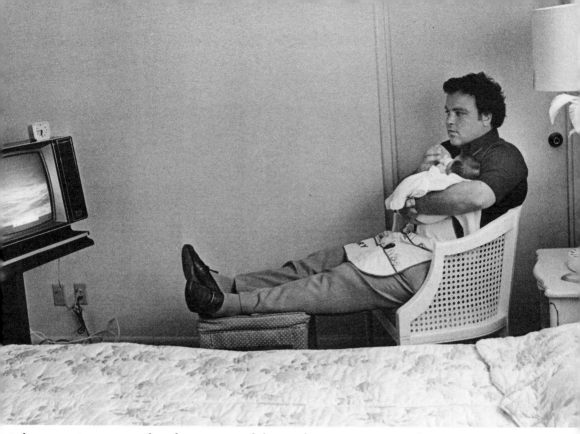

Infant care is a twenty-four hour responsibility and requires team work.
(Alison Ehrlich Wachstein, from Pregnant Moments, Morgan & Morgan,
1978)

endless worries and self-doubt of the depressed patient, but, in the end,
it is the people at home who help the most. They offer the mother sorely
needed relief from a situation that feels like a nightmare so she can recuperate and regain her perspective. They encourage her to go out of
the house for the day, help her rest by getting up for the baby at night.
If she's breast-feeding, they respect that and wake her for feeding, then
take over baby care again. The supportive home environment that helps
a woman get over her depression is no different from the mothering
experiences recommended for all new mothers as they learn infant feeding (see chapter 8). With that kind of solid support in the first place, it's
unlikely that a woman will end up in postpartum depression.

Once in the situation, however, I encourage husbands to use their
imaginations to help their wives get back on their feet. When possible,
they should follow the mother's lead, rather than telling her what to do.
They should encourage her self-confidence rather than question her
judgment and capabilities. The goal is to help her function as well as she
can, not as well as her husband or family think she should. Here are some
unusual ways in which husbands helped:

"My husband used to sit next to me and feed me dinner while I fed the baby. I know it sounds crazy, but he was giving me the strength to be a mother."

"My husband bought a used Ping-Pong table and set it up in the basement. We played Ping-Pong with the tears running down my cheeks."

Ping-Pong and hand-feeding the mother, to my mind, are a lot better medicine than tranquilizers, shock treatment, or institutionalization. Any of these may become necessary if the situation is acute enough, but if early signs of distress are responded to with constructive help, a full-blown breakdown can often be avoided. Love and acceptance of the mother, easy communication of feelings, and sufficient help are the best preventives.

Florida-based Dr. Richard Gordon, a psychiatrist, and his wife Katherine were able to halve the incidence of postpartum depression in a prepared group of mothers, as compared to a comparable group they did not teach, by conducting a class based on certain fundamental principles. Their work was done almost two decades ago, but their mental health checklist still provides a sound structure to protect the new mother emotionally.

Mental Health Checklist for New Mothers

(adapted from the work of Gordon and Gordon)

1. The responsibilities of motherhood are learned. *GET INFORMED.*
2. Get help from your husband and dependable friends and relatives.
3. Make friends with "experienced" couples.
4. Don't overload yourself with unimportant tasks.
5. Don't move soon after the baby arrives.
6. Don't be overconcerned with keeping up appearances.
7. Get plenty of rest and sleep.
8. Don't be a nurse to relatives and others in this period.
9. Confer and consult with your husband, your friends, and your family.DISCUSS YOUR PLANS AND WORRIES.
10. Don't give up outside interests, but cut down on your responsibilities and rearrange your schedule.
11. Arrange for baby-sitters early.
12. Get a family doctor early.

Another vital way to keep the stresses of new motherhood from escalating into an emotional breakdown is to arrange for company and communication with other women after the baby comes. To the dismay of mental health professionals who stress this point, most pregnant women continue to rely on their husbands for companionship until the last minute and never think about whom they will be socializing with during the day when their husbands are back to work. In the first weeks, they feel completely isolated with the new baby, and then, when they do venture forth into the world with a baby carriage, they feel adrift in a sea of strangers.

Don't underestimate the problems you're likely to face in finding a compatible group of new friends once you are a mother. It has been shown that:

1. New mothers who begin postpartum programs in the first few weeks after childbirth get the most out of them and have an easier time adjusting to motherhood than those who delay starting.

2. Women who have made arrangements to start postpartum programs while they're pregnant find it easier to start going out than those who wait to find the groups after the baby is born.

The next, and final chapter of this book will help you find the best community programs available as you are recuperating and adjusting to the baby. You will be surprised to find how many exciting possibilities there are.

14

Finding Support in the Community

Now is the time to reach out and find friends in the community who will be there to help and advise you as you are becoming a parent. Unless you're one of the very few people in the United States who live in a cross-generational family or with other young, child-rearing couples, you will need to go out into the community to locate these necessary supports. Making casual friends at the supermarket or in the park is not as good; what you need is a setting where people can be open and honest and not keep up a false front, where they are willing to communicate feelings, problems, and solutions.

After childbirth, most women crave the company of other women; they want to chat about all the fascinating details of their new lives: How many hours did the baby sleep last night? Do your stitches still hurt when you have sex? Is ointment or cream better for a cracked nipple? What if the baby wants to nurse for hours? What are you going to do about your stretch marks? How do you play with a one-month-old baby? Isn't it strange how your baby seems to understand every word you say?

Elisabeth Bing has learned in her many years of experience helping young mothers that what women want is to exchange experiences with other women. "There is hardly room for the professional," she says. I concur. The most helpful facilities are those run by and for mothers themselves, with professionals taking a back seat.

Hospitals, social-work agencies, child-guidance and psychotherapy clinics offer classes for new mothers in "community outreach" programs. Several of these classes are outstanding, directed by top mental health professionals, but unfortunately, others are used as training grounds for young, inexperienced leaders. In some settings, there are only one or two classes—a lecture on infant development and a demonstration of postpartum exercises. This is only a cosmetic approach. False reassurances and a smattering of information are hardly sufficient for new mothers.

I must admit I also take a somewhat jaundiced view of another kind of professional service that is being offered to new mothers. This is the postpartum discussion group with a professional social worker or psychologist as leader, offered at an attractively low fee to middle-class people by private child-guidance or psychotherapy centers. One of the major motives of these agencies is to attract patients to therapy. That subtly changes the focus from consolidating people's strengths to exploiting their weaknesses, and, I believe, is taking unfair advantage of women at a vulnerable stage in their lives. If these community clinics really want to promote the mental health of new parents, they should spend the time and effort to train mothers to work as peer counselors and group facilitators, rather than running groups themselves.

Any group led by an "expert" encourages dependency rather than personal strength. There are times when a new mother needs to be dependent, when she needs to be mothered. This temporary dependency can be turned to advantage if the information being imparted is imbedded in a parental kind of relationship, like The School for Mothering (discussed later in the chapter). But when a woman really needs a friend, not a mother or a father figure, she shouldn't be encouraged to buy that friendship from a doctor.

Women must learn to relate to obstetricians, pediatricians, and psychotherapists as knowledgeable consumers, not dependent children. I have seen too many expert-led groups turn to the leader for the "right" answer, for approval, for acceptance—even for affection. It is a seductive scene for all—including the professional—but not nearly so ego-strengthening as good peer help and support, and the encouragement to look *inside* for the right answers.

MOTHERS' GROUPS

The largest number of self-help support groups available throughout the country are offered by childbirth education organizations that are members of ICEA. ASPO, which originally organized only to prepare mothers in the Lamaze method of natural childbirth, is now expanding its program to include postpartum discussion groups and exercise groups. It's a good idea to call the state coordinators of *both* organizations because they don't exchange lists. You may be referred to a group in your locale that has only a "hot-line" for emergencies and no course. Some communities have ongoing "coffees" to which all new mothers are welcome. And still other communities have regular ongoing classes. At the time of this writing, more than two hundred groups are actively meeting.

Groups usually go four to six sessions. Eight to ten mothers come—with their babies during the day or with their husbands at night. The women give and get ideas and expert information about baby care, typical reactions after childbirth, sexual readjustment, family planning, feeding the baby, infant development, relating to the pediatrician, training baby-sitters, first aid and safety—and any other matter that concerns a member of the group.

The best classes offer co-leadership by two trained "group facilitators" who have taken leadership training classes. In many communities, experts in pediatrics, nutrition, social work, and psychology help train these peer counselors and leaders. They learn how to teach in an easygoing way, giving class members plenty of time to express their feelings and concerns.

Peggy Drake, former director of teacher services for ICEA nationally, encourages all new mothers to join one of the groups. She says, "You really do need to find some people who are in the same boat as you are, having the same experiences. It helps you know that you are normal."

There is no "model" course or group. Each one is developed by individuals who meet needs as best they can, with the help and training offered by the national organization. The following descriptions of three separate courses will give you an idea of the range of possibilities.

Gay Courter, a filmmaker, helped to organize the postpartum program in northern New Jersey. After her first child was born, her local childbirth teacher helped her enormously and she learned how much all new mothers need support and help. This inspired her to help others in turn. Here is how the program she helped to develop is working:

Women in northern New Jersey preregister for four postpartum classes when they sign up for eight natural childbirth preparation classes through the childbirth education association in the area. All twelve classes cost $30, and, because they're paid for in advance, women manage to get to postpartum groups shortly after their babies come. Before the system was devised, Gay says, it was hard to get women to come.

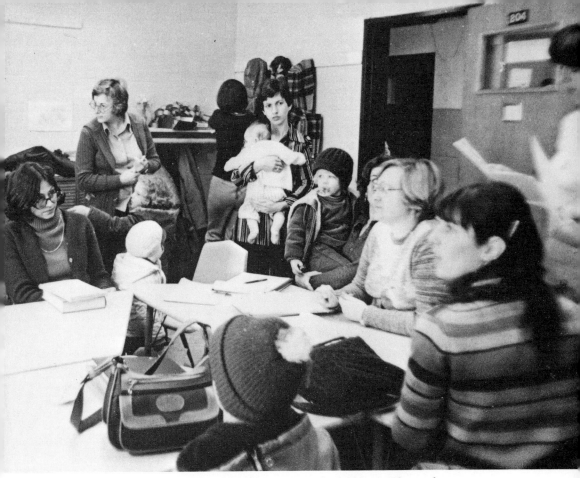

*At the unique Mothers' Center in Hicksville, New York, active mothers plan
exciting programs of mutual support and education. (Courtesy of The
Mother's Center, United Methodist Church, Hicksville, N.Y.)*

"They were afraid to drive, or afraid to appear stupid—there were a variety of reasons."

Classes meet in "volunteer homes" of former members whose children are now older. These hostesses greet the mothers, prepare refreshments, etc., and have the opportunity to watch two co-leaders in action. Often this inspires them to take the leadership training course themselves.

It's an interesting phenomenon that once a new mother's baby is a little older, she feels the need to help others. Some women prefer to become active in community efforts to improve hospital facilities. Others want to communicate to others what they have learned. Opportunities to satisfy either inclination are offered by all the childbirth education groups, and they welcome new mothers to their growing ranks.

The New Jersey groups are run with great sensitivity. New mothers are never put in the position of having to vie for attention with leaders' children, for example. Two leaders work together so that mothers can perceive, from the start, that there is no one "right" way to solve a problem. Leaders are trained not to impose their own values, and women of every level of education and station of life find a lot in common and can relate comfortably in this democratic atmosphere.

Quite a different course is being offered on Long Island, in New York, under ASPO sponsorship. In this class, the emphasis is on the practicalities of baby care. For $10, mothers are offered a six-session course. A movie is shown, experts in psychology and child care are invited to speak, there is classroom demonstration and discussion, and plenty of time left over for socialization.

In Seattle, Washington, the Parenthood Education Program (member of ICEA) offers two classes. One is for parents of newborns and children up to two years, and the second is for toddlers. Discussed are child-guidance techniques, safety and first aid, food and nutrition (for the younger group—introducing solids, weaning, etc.), child development, and "play and toy opportunities for the child." For the parents of older children, child-guidance techniques are introduced to prevent or reduce conflict. Discussions are held to prepare children to deal with fear and death and to begin to understand moral values.

POSTPARTUM EXERCISE CLASSES

Many women regularly attend exercise or dance classes before they're pregnant and are just itching to get back afterward. I will not need to tell them of the pleasures of rhythmic exercise and its great rewards.

It's important not to let overeagerness get in the way of good judgment when you begin postpartum exercises, however. You can begin the postpartum rehabilitation and pelvic floor exercises described in chapter 2 in the hospital, but you should wait for your six-week checkup before starting more serious exercising.

Pelvic floor exercises, in fact, can start on the recovery table. Postpartum exercises are carefully graded from day one to help you feel stronger and more secure each day.

At the end of six weeks, you can go to a dance-exercise class and feel that your body finally belongs to you again! For breast-feeders, this feeling is particularly important. Socialization and regular commitment to a class are ego-strengtheners, too.

However, I caution you to select a teacher who is experienced in helping new mothers. Because of the hormones you secrete during pregnancy, all your ligaments will be softened for up to seven months after the baby's birth. It is safer to exercise under the guidance of a professional teacher with a good knowledge of the anatomy and physiology of pregnancy, labor, and delivery.

Your childbirth teacher or La Leche leader should know of a good local class. She may even teach a class herself, in partnership with professional dance instructors, whose pregnant students often sign up for postpartum classes before the baby comes.

LA LECHE LEAGUE

This is the largest, most successful self-help group of mothers in the world. Started by seven breast-feeding women in 1956 to provide mutual support at a time when breast-feeding was almost "a lost art" in America, it now reaches more than a million women a year through group meetings, correspondence, telephone help, and the league journal.

The basic manual of the organization has sold more than 600,000 copies in the present edition. There also are numerous leaflets, pamphlets, and books available from the Illinois office about prenatal care and childbirth, breast-feeding, child care, and the family, the La Leche League itself, nutrition, and the psychological aspects of the mother-child relationship.

That American women are returning to breast-feeding is due, in good measure, to the League's efforts. We still have the lowest rate of breast-feeders in the world, and Mary Cossman of the La Leche League of Great Neck, New York, maintains that "It's still hard for a young, inexperienced woman to find substantial support for her breast-feeding outside of La Leche." It's not only for breast-feeding help that a woman should join La Leche. Mrs. Cossman says, "I became interested in La Leche because they speak for the children . . . helpless creatures. Who is speaking for their rights? I nurse my babies not as a method of feeding, but as a way of mothering." Mrs. Cossman spends a great deal of her free time helping other women. "If we women don't help one another, who is going to help us?" she says. While she speaks for herself, she also reflects the basic attitudes of the organization—good mothering and good comradeship among women.

League members inspire one another, support one another, advise one another—even give milk to one another's babies when necessary. A La Leche group consists of ten to fifteen women who meet in one mother's home on a regular basis in the evening. Babies are welcomed as necessary, and dues are voluntary. Between meetings, the leaders are available for telephone consultation and problem-solving on a day-to-day basis. Here is the leadership philosophy, as expressed by Mrs. Cossman: "We don't look for a perfect solution, just successful functioning. Everyone is entitled to be different. We just share experiences."

The organization officially frowns on formula supplements and early solids, however, so try not to feel overwhelmed if you can't meet their standards. Many women are unwilling or unable to make a commitment to total, long-range breast-feeding and want to be "partial lactators" only. They may not breast-feed as long or as completely as others in their La Leche group, but they also need its support. Often, by the time the next baby comes along, they're more comfortable with motherhood and ready to breast-feed longer. The La Leche leader and the group are there to help each mother achieve her own goals.

For referral to the group nearest you: Write to La Leche League, International, 9616 Minneapolis Avenue, Franklin Park, Illinois 60131.

A SCHOOL FOR MOTHERING

There is very little opportunity today to prepare for mothering in a natural way—by observing experienced mothers with their children and helping them with baby care. After the baby comes, many women find, to their surprise, that they feel physically clumsy and alienated from their baby. They're afraid to pick him up and hold him, unsure if they will ever learn to soothe and satisfy him.

One reason mothers want their babies to stuff themselves with milk and sleep for long stretches is that then they will not have to face these unhappy feelings of anxiety and inadequacy. They wish they had someplace to go where an expert could observe them with the baby, listen to his cries, watch him move, and interpret what is going on.

For mothers with these feelings, the seventy or more research centers now studying mother-infant interaction and teaching mothers to respond kinesthetically to their babies may be just the right community resource. Some centers are operated by child psychiatrists belonging to the American Academy of Child Psychiatry, and others are under the direction of specialists in adult psychiatry and clinical psychology. Unfortunately, the American Academy of Child Psychiatry is unwilling to act as a central referral source because it doesn't wish to imply approval of any programs that are still being developed. You'll have to ask your pediatrician or obstetrician if there's a research center in your community, or inquire at your local hospital, medical school, or university.

One center has been in operation in Port Washington, New York, for about six years, under the direction of Dr. Judith Kestenberg, psychoanalyst and child psychiatrist, and of Arnhilt Buelte, movement specialist. The name of the center is "Center for Parents and Children." It is operating under the auspices of a non-profit organisation, called "Child Development Research." Its number is 516-883-3850 or -7135.

Despite the formidable name, the center provides a creative learning *and* playing experience for pregnant women and new mothers. The founders and directors, Dr. Kestenberg and Mrs. Buelte probably are more movement-oriented than most other researchers. They are dedicated to helping parents heighten their body sensitivity during pregnancy and in parenthood, have developed fine diagnostic tools to spot problem areas, and teach parents through direct, physical demonstrations that are far easier to understand than the verbiage of many other child-care experts and psychological consultants.

Two groups meet regularly (for location inquire at 516-883-7135); one for mothers and children aged two to four, the second for mothers with infants and toddlers up to two, fathers and anyone who is intimately connected with the child. If a mother in the older group has a new baby, she can bring the baby along so that the older sibling can express his concerns and make a better adjustment.

For the older children, there is an art and movement program, free and organized play. Parents participate as assistant teachers until the children are comfortable enough to stay on their own. The younger group meets two mornings a week for two hours. Then everyone has lunch together, after which there is free play and a delightful "music relationship session" where mothers and babies sing homemade songs and move about to guitar and piano music. Mothers keep a journal of their day-to-day activities, questions, and concerns, and these are responded to in writing by the staff. The cost is about $200 for the younger group and $325 for the older and $30.00 for the parents' evening course, and the participants get a good deal

In the "baby orchestra" at the Child Development Research Center in Port Washington, New York, the newborn to two-year-olds develop a sense of identity. (Courtesy of Dr. Judith Kestenberg, The Center for Parents and Children, Child Development Research Center, Sands Point, N.Y.)

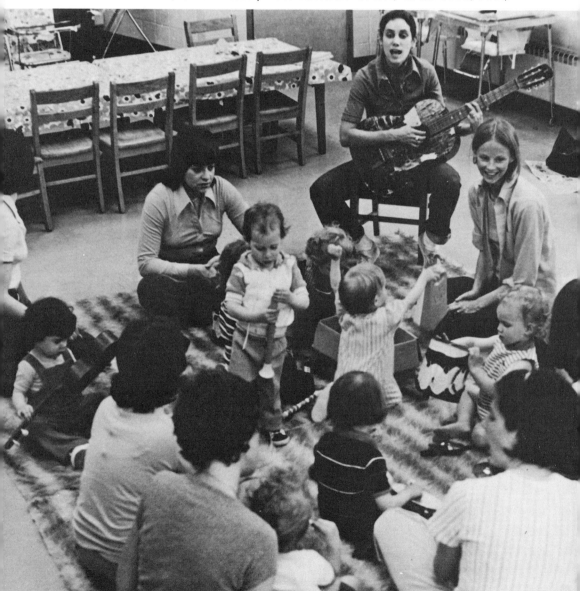

of personal help for their money. In the best tradition of educating new mothers, it includes a good bit of mothering for the mother, too.

The entire staff (all volunteers except the teacher) were busy interacting with and stimulating the young babies' group on the day I visited. Dr. Kestenberg, energetic and grandmotherly, was showing the mother of a three-month-old how to hold the bottle more flexibly, moving it in and out a bit in response to the baby's breathing. She pointed out how the baby looked into the mother's eyes, how his hands reached out to hold and caress her body while he sucked. Meanwhile, other little babies were crawling up and down a safe carpeted staircase especially constructed for them. Later, in the center of the room, a young teacher played the guitar and sang a song describing what each baby was doing at the moment. Mothers clapped happily, sang, moved in time to the rhythms. Even the babies seemed to be banging their toy instruments in time to the music. "How do you like the baby orchestra?" asked a beaming Dr. Kestenberg.

Pregnant women are invited to come to these mothers' groups to observe and play with the babies. They have their own course of exercises in the evening. In some situations, with the obstetrician's consent, Dr. Kestenberg even attends a mother's labor and delivery. Afterward, she communicates her observations of the newborn to the parents in an office consultation. That is truly a unique service.

This facility is different from any other and depends on the guiding force of people like Dr. Kestenberg, Arnhilt Buelte, Estelle Borowitz, Dr. Marcus, and Elaine Schnee. Like the wise grandmother of old, Dr. Kestenberg has the accumulated wisdom of the tribe and delights in passing it on.

POSTPARTUM—A GROWTH EXPERIENCE

More people are reaching out for help from mental health experts *before* they have serious problems. This is called "preventive mental health." Some psychiatrists, psychologists, social workers, and childbirth experts are responding by forming "holistic health centers" that don't treat sick people but teach normal ones to deal more effectively with the complexities and stresses of everyday life.

Some of these holistic health centers specialize in family life, particularly the stressful time of new parenthood. Since the movement is very

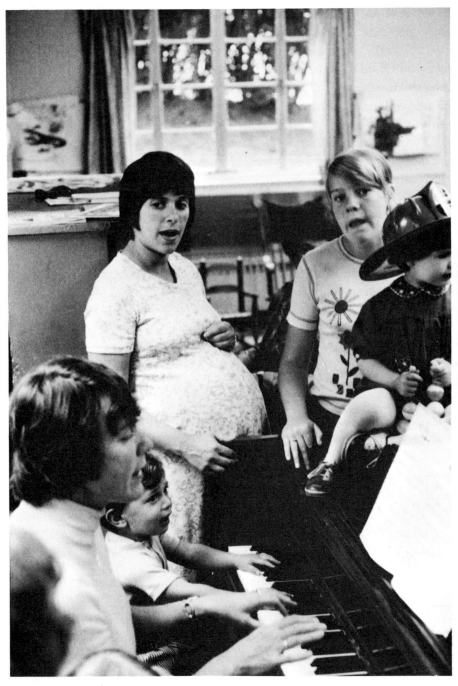

Pregnant women have the rare opportunity to interact with experienced mothers and their babies at Dr. Kestenberg's Long Island "School for Mothering." (Courtesy of Dr. Judith Kestenberg, The Center for Parents and Children, Child Development Research Center, Sands Point, N.Y.)

new, there aren't many centers around the country. Several facilities in New York and California can serve as models of what can be done.

In Cotati, California, the Center for Family Growth offers courses that focus on childbirth and family life as an opportunity for psycho-spiritual growth. It has a rich, imaginative curriculum (described in chapter 7, under "Yogic Childbirth") that will appeal to those who share its spiritual philosophy.

The Holistic Childbirth Preparation and Family Center of New York, at 373 Westminster Road, in Brooklyn, New York 11226, has attractively packaged and priced courses that are designed to meet all the needs of new parents: Health Care during Pregnancy; Preparation for Childbirth through Lamaze and other Methods; Baby Care and Breast-feeding; Marital and Sexual Changes; From the Amazing Newborn to Toddler; Nutrition; and Movement for Health and Fun.

The Family Institute of Berkeley, at 1542 LeRoy Avenue in Berkeley, California, offers an interesting eight-week experiential course called Becoming Parents. "It assists expectant couples and new parents to make appropriate maturational transitions so they can be more comfortable and successful in their new role as parents as well as maintaining the strength of their bond as a couple. . . . The essence of the workshop is the communication between husband and wife of similarities and differences of needs, wants, and expectations in relation to parenthood." This course is being taught to mental health professionals who will return to work in their own communities, and it may be available in a hospital, community center, or university in your area.

People who have participated in "growth experiences"—marriage encounters, adult education extension programs, and the like—know that these courses can be inspiring, informative, and a lot of fun. They do not appeal to everyone, but if you are interested, I can recommend such a course as a valuable preparation for new parenthood.

THE MOTHERS' CENTER—A NEW MODEL

For many years, England and the Commonwealth countries have had a tradition of "mothercraft"—teaching inexperienced women the home-making, child-care, and home-nursing skills they will need as mothers. Usually, these are taught in local community centers so women have a friendly place to go with their new babies as well as to get help with practical skills.

A community center for new mothers is still a very new idea in America, but it is about the best idea I know to provide the emotional support and practical help that has been lost in our society where geographical mobility and small, isolated family units have become the norm and the traditional strong ties to relatives and neighbors no longer exist.

Our American model, the Mothers' Center in Hicksville, Long Island (located at the United Methodist Church on Old Country Road and Nelson Avenue; tel.: 822-4539), barely resembles the English one. The program does include preparing for childbirth and first aid and informal help with breast-feeding, but primarily it consists of community and center projects and of discussion groups that deal in depth with many aspects of the mother-child and family relationships. Women are helped to work out problems that developed during childbirth and to replace old attitudes of dependency on experts and competitiveness with other women with self-reliance and mutual respect.

The Mothers' Center is an important advance in preventive mental health. Its concepts are attracting a good deal of attention from experts, and most importantly, from mothers in other sections of the country. Here are the names and addresses of three more Mothers' Centers that have opened recently, based on the original model and with the assistance and guidance of the first group of mothers:

The Mothers' Center of Suffolk County
73 Glen Summer Road
Holbrook, New York 11741
Contact Dale Doyle

The Mothers' Center of St. Louis
3955 Camelot Estates Court
St. Louis, Missouri 63129
Contact Resa Workman

The Mothers' Center of Rockland County
33 West Hickory Street
Spring Valley, New York 10977
Contact Jill Lagnado

The first Mothers' Center started with the help of the Family Service Association of Nassau and the United Methodist Church, plus small donations and a small grant from the North Shore Unitarian Church.

It is open three days a week, from 9:30 to 2:30, and any mother can join. The membership donation is $10 per year. There are two large, excellently equipped child-care rooms—one for infants and one for toddlers—and the center pays a child-care staff to provide a stable, ongoing relationship for the youngsters. It closes for the summer and opens each fall with new groups, planned in response to the expressed interests of members. Each group has a maximum of ten mothers plus two center-trained "group facilitators" or discussion leaders, and meets for seven sessions. There are four new programs each season.

Last year's program included discussion of delivery experiences, childbirth preparation, development and care of infants and toddlers, special problems with adopted children, and relationship issues with school-age children. There were mothers' groups, fathers' groups, couples' groups, first-aid classes, and lectures by visiting childbirth and child-rearing experts. Maternity and children's clothes were recycled, a film was produced, research was continued, and new research plans made. Some mothers were referred to appropriate community resources for help with problems that needed professional attention.

The Mothers' Center has researched the services of each hospital in the community and arranged for the results to be printed in the local newspaper. In some hospitals, they have arranged to conduct tours for expectant parents and have participated in the renovation and decoration of a new maternity wing in a local hospital. They have been influential in improving family-centered facilities in other hospitals and maintain excellent cooperative relationships with all doctors and hospitals in the area.

The Mothers' Center offers an innovative "peer counselor" program. Anyone who is interested can learn ego psychology, counseling techniques, and group dynamics. Professionals in the community come in to help out, but that program, like everything else at the Mothers' Center, is firmly in the hands of the women.

Open involvement and lack of status differences is the philosophy of the Mothers' Center. All members can sit in on all meetings—whether they're executive or administrative, peer counseling, self-help discussions, or community projects. There is no hierarchy among the mothers, and professionals are welcome to offer their expertise but not allowed to take over. Mothers are in charge, and they jealously guard their autonomy and independence. "We try to build self-esteem and give knowledge so that every woman can trust herself to make the best decision—for herself—all the way through."

No one point of view about childbirth or mothering practices is advocated—not natural childbirth, not breast-feeding. Group leaders are careful to discourage peer pressure in the group discussions and "never presume to give medical information."

I watched a group called "Mothers and Daughters" in action. Nine mothers, two "facilitators," and one baby were present. The mothers were surprisingly conservative in their manner and appearance. I had expected more activism, more anger, more deviance. Instead, I saw a group of nicely dressed, decorous young women who might have been sitting in the neighborhood playground watching their children.

They didn't relate as women do in the playground, however, comparing their babies' weight gain and sleep schedules. The facilitators started things off with a few skillful questions, and soon women were discussing day-to-day problems and sharing past history with refreshing openness.

My impression was that these women know exactly where they stand and what they want out of their lives at present. They want to be mothers, full time. They are tolerant and accepting of other points of view and of women who want to live differently, but they resent having their preferences devalued, of being made defensive about staying home while their children are small. It may well be that in a decade these same women will be in another kind of discussion group, preparing to go back to work. For the time being, however, they want the comradeship and approval of other women like themselves, who are committed to full-time maternity.

I was enormously impressed with the quality of the discussion in this peer-led group. No one looked to the facilitators for approval or for answers. They related freely, as equals. This is quite different from professionally-led groups. In that setting, the women had a tendency to revert to the role of submissive, argumentative, or competitive children who view the leader as a good or bad "mama." The peer-group experience is far more ego-strengthening, much superior.

AN IDEAL:
FROM MOTHERS' CENTER TO WOMEN'S CENTER

One day the philosophy of the Mothers' Center will be incorporated into a Woman's Center that will give support and information to women as they move from adolescence to old age. Included would be groups for teenagers on sex, childbirth, and baby care; childbirth preparation classes for pregnant women; parents' groups and mothers' groups for every age and special child; single women's groups; marriage groups; groups to help with menopause and old age; sex information and therapy for adults; and lectures by professionals in all mental and physical health areas. Even "homelike deliveries" could be part of such a Women's Center, if it were located near a hospital.

Already there are many women's health groups all over the country working toward fulfilling these ideals. There may be one in your own area. HealthRight, a women's health education and advocacy group at 175 Fifth Avenue, New York, New York 10010, has an up-to-date file and will be happy to refer you to the one closest to your home. HealthRight also writes, produces, and distributes literature dealing with health and the health-care system and teaches courses for women in these areas. It has a unique quarterly newsletter (you can subscribe to it for $5 a year), that links groups and resources. Recent issues have dealt with such concerns as infant malnutrition in the third world, battered women, the effects of hormones on mothers and unborn babies, and home birth.

CREATE YOUR OWN BEST CHILDBIRTH EXPERIENCE

Your childbirth experience will go more smoothly and successfully if you:

Become aware of the current social and medical scene, the cultural pressures we all face, the economic realities.

Get informed about your feelings so you can arrange for the type of childbirth preparation that is right for you.

Get involved so you can find the right doctor and hospital or childbirth setting for you.

Get support for your postpartum period *before* the baby comes.

Keep in mind that different types of personalities respond to different methods of delivery, different settings, different style of doctoring. The doctor can act as your advocate with the hospital if he or she chooses to. Hospitals will bend their rules. Remember that you are buying services that doctors and hospitals want to sell.

Emotional support after delivery is important to prevent postpartum breakdown, which is a very common, though not often serious, form of depression. Find a group of women, either on your own or through one of the recommended services, who will build you up, not play on your weaknesses and fears. Any good postpartum service or doctor will refer you for professional help if that is what you need.

Get help with postpartum depression if your symptoms last more than a week, if you're crying uncontrollably, feel despairing, overwhelmed, seriously rejecting of the baby, or unable to function on a day-to-day basis. Brief counseling can be very effective to get you and your family back on the right track.

When you go for help with your emotional problems, be a knowledgeable consumer, just as you have been advised to be when selecting your obstetrician and pediatrician. You must feel positive that the counselor is empathetic with you and knowledgeable about the realities you are facing. Avoid the authoritarian figure—this type got you into your fix in the first place!

The chances are very good that you won't need professional help for emotional problems if you follow the suggestions in this book to create your own best childbirth experience.

Resources that orchestrate "the natural way," "sisterhood," and expert advice are increasingly available. You'll be glad you're having a baby now, in the seventies, in the United States of America. Good luck!

(Dr. David Kliot/Brookdale Hospital Medical Center)

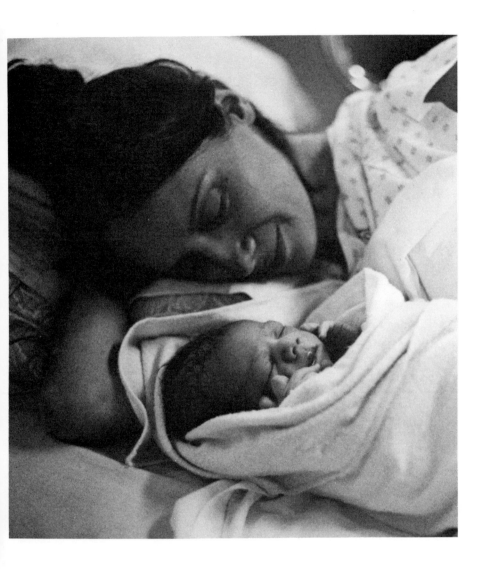

Appendix I: ICEA Province/State Coordinators

Canadian Region

Alberta: Elaine Montgomery, 8207 10th St., SW, Calgary T2V 1M7

British Columbia: Louise Mangan, 2835 Revelstoke Court, UBC V6T 1N8

Manitoba: Beverly and Thomas Lampman, 1132 Clarence Ave., Winnipeg R3T 1S9

New Brunswick: Barbara Palmer, RR 3, Hillsborough, EOA 1X0

North West Territories: Nancy Menagh, Box 2471, Yellowknife X0E 1H0

Nova Scotia: Joella and Jim Foulds, RR #1, Bras D'Or B0C 1BO

Ontario: Margaret Falkenhagen, 49 Woodhill Crescent, Ottawa K1B 3B7

Prince Edward Island: Kerstin Martin, RR #2, Bonshaw C0A 1C0

Quebec: Lynda and Gilbert McElroy, 47 Saratoga, Aylmer J9H 4A5

Saskatchewan: Phyllis Wilson, Box 97, Dubuc S0Z 0R0

Yukon Territory: Donna Wilkinson, 7 Ketza Road, Whitehorse Y1A 2C6

U.S. Eastern Region

Connecticut: Barbara Soderberg, 59 Slocum Road, Hebron 06248

Delaware: Roger and Terry Sipress, 1709 Wembley Dr., Wilmington 19809

Maine: Penny Bohac, RFD 1, Box 11-C, Brooks 04921

Maryland & DC: Jayne Fedowitz, 11393 Bantry Terrace, Fairfax, VA 22030

Massachusetts: Bonnie Donovan, Camp Parker, Pembroke 02359

New Hampshire: Betty Foster, 39 Hickory Dr., Amherst 03031

New Jersey: Jean Levine, 902 Oak Ave., Linwood 08221

New York City & Long Island: Marguerite Perinelli, 587 Greeley Ave., Staten Island 10306

New York: Vivien Wiesner, 1826 Western Ave., Albany 12203

Pennsylvania: Dave and Glenda Erskine, 912 S. Park Ave., Glensaw 15116

Rhode Island: Cory Fink, 422 Wayland Ave., Providence 02906

Vermont: Debi Ginsburgh, P.O. Box 423, Bellows Falls 05101

U.S. Southern Region

Alabama: Fran Harrison, Rt 5, Box 234, Decatur 35603

Arkansas: Judy Yeager, 1118 Wild Turkey Court, Little Rock 72211

Florida: Laurie Goodrich, 1966 Ezelle Ave., NE, Largo 33540

Georgia: Marie and Ron Reed, 218 Montego Circle, Riverdale 30274

Kentucky: Katherine Johnson, 1941 Deerwood Ave., Louisville 40205

Louisiana: Marion and Mike Donohoe, 376 Markham, Slidell 70458

Mississippi: Lisa Walcott, 1037 Ceder St., Greenville 38701

North Carolina: Debra Patterson, 507 Blueridge Rd., Carrboro 27510

Oklahoma: Cara Ditto, 218 Stanton Dr., Norman 73071

South Carolina: Carol Pinckney, Fairfied, McClellanville 29458

Tennessee: Sharon Lee Annis, 869-AW. Outer Dr. Oak Ridge 37830

Texas: Susan Mansur, 2433 Bridge, Abilene 79603

Virginia: Lynn Thye, 804 Draper Road, Blacksburg 24060

West Virginia: Janet Nemeschy, 10 Mt. Vista Dr., Buckhannon 26201

U.S. Midwestern Region

Illinois: Judy Knobloch, RR2, Box 120, Wyoming 61491

Indiana: Paula Cockrum, 6615 Kratzville Rd., Evansville 47710

Iowa: Katie Keefer, 929 Idaho, Davenport 52804

Kansas: Vionetta Schmidt, 320 North 15th, Manhattan 66502

Michigan: (upper) Jeanne Rose, 1711 Lake Shore Dr., Macanaba 49829

Michigan: (lower) Kathe Mantyla, 2189 C Meadowlawn, Holt 48842

Minnesota: Ann Peirce, 12135 24th Ave. N., Minneapolis 55441

Missouri: Marion Gould, 10919 Campbell, Kansas City 64131

Nebraska: Penny Enyeart, 507 W. 9th St., North Platte 69101

Ohio: Linda and David Bailey, 2183 Larchdale Ave., Cuyahoga Falls 44221

South Dakota: Donna Larson, 3913 E. Seventh St., Sioux Falls 57103

Wisconsin: Carol Fowler, 1016 Van Buren St., Madison 53711

U.S. Western Region

Alaska: Jeannette Seale, Route 3, Box 3827, Juneau 99801

Arizona: Margery Simchak, 14245 North 19th Ave., Phoenix 85023

California: (north) Lynda Bachelor, 236 Tunisia, Fort Ord 93941

California: (south) Joyce Hull, 4412 48th Street, San Diego 92115

Colorado: Jayne Polliard, 15 East Columbia Street, Colorado Springs 80907

Hawaii: Dawn Morell, 107 East 2nd Street, Hickam AFB 96818

Idaho: Patty Neville, 1045 North Aruther, Pocatello 83201

Montana: Alice Marie Emond, Route 1, Box 5A, Lewistown 59457

Nevada: Geri Rentchler, 1201 South Rancho Dr., Las Vegas 89102

New Mexico: Bill and Susan Prim, 1702 Callehon Cordelia, Santa Fe 87501

Oregon: Julie Thomas, 2845 Greentree Way, Eugene 97402

Utah: Sherri Smart, 450 West 500 South, Tooele 84074

Washington (east) Ginny Gagner, 9611 East 10th, Spokane 99206

Washington (west) Leah Gray, 4521 113th Place NE, Marysville 98270

Wyoming: Barbara Sullivan, 3521 Capital Ave., Cheyeene 82007

Appendix II: ASPO
State Coordinators

Alabama
ASPO of Central Alabama
516 East Fairview Avenue
Montgomery, AL 36106

Arizona
Arizona South Central ASPO
c/o Karen Hernandez
2201 West Emerald Circle
Mesa, AZ 85202

California
Bay Area ASPO
P.O. Box 6112
Elmwood Station
Berkeley, CA 94705

ASPO of Los Angeles
1543 West Olympic Boulevard
Suite 343
Los Angeles, CA 90015

Delaware
Delmarva ASPO
712 Burning Tree Circle
Salisbury, MD 21801

District of Columbia
Washington, D.C. Area ASPO
1411 K Street, NW
Washington, D.C. 20005

Illinois
Northern Illinois ASPO
P.O. Box 174
Highland Park, IL 60035

Louisiana
ASPO on the Bayou
402 Harwell Drive
Lafayette, LA 70503

Maryland
See *Delaware* and *District of
Columbia*

New Jersey
Central New Jersey ASPO
201 Great Hills Road
Bridgewater, NJ 08807

Greater Camden Area ASPO
P.O. Box 223
Moorestown, NJ 08057

Monmouth-Ocean ASPO
P.O. Box 171
Keyport, NJ 07735

Northern New Jersey ASPO
P.O. Box 562
Ridgewood, NJ 07450

Princeton Area ASPO
289 Bolton Road
East Windsor, NJ 08520

New York
Long Island ASPO
266 Asharoken Avenue
Northport, NY 11768

Mid-Hudson ASPO
P.O. Box 506
Fishkill, NY 12524

New York City ASPO
P.O. Box 725
Midtown Station
New York, NY 10018

Niagara Frontier ASPO
P.O. Box 1642
Buffalo, NY 14216

Westchester ASPO
P.O. Box 125
Scarborough
Briarcliff Manor, NY 10510

North Carolina
Charlotte ASPO
P.O. Box 9547
Charlotte, NC 28299

Foothills ASPO
P.O. Drawer 1508
Morgantown, NC 28655

Oregon
Lane County ASPO
P.O. Box 5083
Eugene, OR 97405

Pennsylvania
Lamaze Educators of
Southeastern
Pennsylvania
P.O. Box 27250
Philadelphia, PA 19118

Pennsylvania
Southwestern Pennsylvania
ASPO
P.O. Box 9064
Pittsburgh, PA 15224

Twin Tier ASPO
51 Mann Street
Mansfield, PA 16933

South Carolina
Greater Columbia ASPO
2830 Wilmont Avenue
Columbia, SC 29205

Tennessee
Nashville ASPO
c/o Judy McCoy
1111 Parker Place
Brentwood, TN 37027

Texas
San Angelo Childbirth
Training Association
c/o Candy Cristensen
3917 Inglewood
San Angelo, TX 76901

Virginia
Charlottesville-Albemarle
ASPO
P.O. Box 3484
Charlottesville, VA 22903

Valley ASPO
c/o Aleene Pittman
25 Church Street
Staunton, VA 24401

Peninsula ASPO
P.O. Box 5689
Parkview Station
Newport News, VA 23605

For a referral to a group, certified childbirth educator, or supportive physician in an area not listed above, contact the ASPO National Information and Referral Service, 1523 I Street NW, Washington, D.C. 20005.

Bibliography

About Your Body

LAUERSEN, NIELS and WHITNEY, STEVEN. *It's Your Body: A Woman's Guide to Gynecology.* New York: Grosset & Dunlap, 1978.

LLEWELLYN-JONES, DEREK. *Everywoman: A Gynaecological Guide For Life.* London: Faber and Faber, 1973.

SEAMAN. BARBARA. *Women and the Crisis in Sex Hormones.* New York: Rawson, 1977.

THE BOSTON WOMEN'S HEALTH BOOK COLLECTIVE. *Our Bodies, Ourselves.* 2nd. edition. New York: Simon and Schuster, 1976.

About Pregnancy: Nutrition, Sex and Exercise

BING, ELISABETH. *Moving Through Pregnancy.* New York: Bobbs-Merrill, 1975.

BING, ELISABETH AND LIBBY COLMAN. *Making Love During Pregnancy.* New York: Bantam Books, 1977.

BREWER, GAIL SFORZA AND TOM BREWER, M.D., *What Every Pregnant Mother Should Know; The Truth About Diet and Drugs in Pregnancy.* New York: Random House, 1977.

DAVIS, ADELLE. *Let's Have Healthy Children.* New York: Signet/New American Library, 1972.

FLANAGAN, GERALDINE L. *The First Nine Months of Life.* New York: Simon & Schuster, 1962.

GOLDBECK, NIKKI AND DAVID. *The Supermarket Handbook.* New York: Signet/New American Library, 1976.

LAPPE, FRANCES MOORE. *Diet For A Small Planet.* New York: Ballantine Books, 1976.

NOBLE, ELIZABETH. *Essential Exercises for the Childbearing Year.* Boston: Houghton Mifflin Co., 1976.

WILLIAMS, PHYLLIS. *Nourishing Your Unborn Child.* New York: Avon Books, 1974.

About Natural Childbirth: Methods and Philosophy

BING, ELISABETH. *Six Practical Lessons For An Easier Childbirth.* New York: Bantam Books, 1972.

BRADLEY, ROBERT A. *Husband Coached Childbirth.* New York: Harper and Row, rev. 1974. (Bradley Method)

CHABON, IRWIN. *Awake and Aware: Participating In Childbirth Through Psychoprophylaxis.* New York: Dell, 1969. (Aspo—Lamaze)

DICK-READ, GRANTLY. *Childbirth Without Fear.* 2nd ed. New York: Harper and Row, 1959.

GAMPER, MARGARET. *Preparation For the Heir Minded.* Glenview, Ill: Midwest Parentcraft Center, 627 Beaver Road, 1976. (Gamper Method)

HAZELL, LESTER. *Commonsense Childbirth.* New York: Berkley Medallion, 1976.

KITZINGER, SHEILA. *Giving Birth: The Parents' Emotions in Childbirth.* New York: Schocken Books, 1977.

KITZINGER, SHEILA. *The Experience of Childbirth.* New York: Pelican/Penguin, 4th ed., 1978.

LEBOYER, FREDERICK. *Birth Without Violence.* New York: Alfred Knopf, 1975. (Leboyer Method)

MEDVIN, JEANNINE PARVATI. *Prenatal Yoga and Natural Birth.* 555 Highland Avenue, Penngrove, Ca. 94951: Freestone Publishing Collective, 1974 (Yogic Childbirth)

TANZER, DEBORAH AND JEAN BLOCK. *Why Natural Childbirth?.* New York: Doubleday and Co., 1972.

WALTON, VICKI E. *Have It Your Way.* Seattle: Henry Philips Publishing Co., 1977 (Pep - Lamaze)

About Interventions and Alternatives

ARMS, SUZANNE, *Immaculate Deception.* New York: Bantam Books, 1975.

BEAN, CONSTANCE. *Labor and Delivery: An Observer's Diary, What You Should Know About Today's Childbirth.* New York: Doubleday, 1977.

BROOKS, TONYA AND LINDA BENNET. *Giving Birth At Home.* Cerritos, California, Box 1219: Association for Childbirth At Home, Int'l., 1976.

DONOVAN, BONNIE AND RUTH ALLEN. *The Cesarean Birth Experience.* New York: Beacon Press, 1977.

HAIRE, DORIS. *The Cultural Warping Of Childbirth.* A special report by the International Childbirth Education Association, 1972, Seattle: ICEA Book Center, P.O. Box 70258.

HAIRE, DORIS AND JOHN. *Implementing Family Centered Maternity Care With a Central Nursery,* 3rd ed., Seattle, Wash: ICEA Book Center, P.O. Box 70258.

H.O.M.E., *Home Oriented Maternity Experience: A Comprehensive Guide to Home Birth.* 511 New York Ave., Takoma Park, Washington, D.C.: H.O.M.E.

McCLEARY, ELLIOTT H. *New Miracles of Childbirth.* New York: Dell, 1974.

STEWART, DAVID AND LEE, (eds). *Safe Alternatives in Childbirth* (Transcription of 1976 NAPSAC conference). Marble Hill, Missouri 63764: Box 267, NAPSAC, 1976.

STEWART, DAVID AND LEE (eds.). *Twenty-First Century Obstetrics Now.* (transcription of 1977 NAPSAC conference), Vols. I and II, Marble Hill, Missouri 63764: Box 267, NAPSAC, 1977.

About Breastfeeding

EIGER, MARVIN S. AND SALLY W. OLDS. *The Complete Book of Breastfeeding.* New York: Workman Publishing Co., Inc., 1972.

PRYOR, KAREN. *Nursing Your Baby.* New York: Pocket Books, 1976.

RAPHAEL, DANA. *The Tender Gift.* New York: Schocken, 1976.

LA LECHE LEAGUE INTERNATIONAL. *The Womanly Art of Breastfeeding.* Franklin Park, Ill: La Leche League, International, 1963.

About Parenting

BRAZELTON, T. BERRY. *Infants and Mothers: Differences in Development.* Boston: Seymour Lawrence Inc., 1969.

CAPLAN, FRANK, ed. *The First Twelve Months of Life,* New York: Grosset & Dunlap, 1973.

FEATHERINGILL, EVE. *How To Be A Successful Mother.* New York: William Morrow and Co., 1964.

FRAIBERG, SELMA. *Every Child's Birthright: In Defense of Mothering.* New York: Basic Books, 1977.

HYMES, JAMES L., JR. *The Child Under Six.* Englewood Cliffs, N.J.: Prentice-Hall, Inc., 1961.

KLAUS, MARSHALL AND JOHN KENNEL. *Maternal-Infant Bonding.* St. Louis: The C.V. Mosby Co., 1976.

MONTAGU, ASHLEY. *Touching*. New York: Perennial Library, Columbia U. Press, 1971.

NEWTON, NILES. *The Family Book of Child Care*. New York: Harper and Row, 1957.

RIBBLE, MARGARET A. *The Rights of Infants*. New York: Signet/New American Library, 1973.

RODZILSKY, MARYLOU AND BARBARA BANAT. *What Now? A Guide For New Parents*. New York: Charles Scribner's Sons, 1975.

SALK, LEE AND RITA KRAMER. *How To Raise A Human Being*. New York: Random House, 1969.

SPOCK, BENJAMIN. *Baby and Child Care*. New York: Pocket Books, rev. ed., 1976.

THEVENIN, TINE. *The Family Bed*. Minneapolis, Minn.: P.O. Box 16004, 1976.

NOTE: Many of these books are at your public library, paperback bookstore or health food store. Two bookstores that specialize in books about the subject, and will mail any book to you, are:

I.C.A.H. Bookstore
P.O. Box 70258, Seattle, Washington 98107
tel: (206) 789-4444

and

A.C.H.I. Bookstore
Sue Crockett
RD 9 - Fair St. Carmel, NY 10512
Tel: (914) 225-7763

Index

About the Author

Dr. Silvia Feldman, married and the mother of three girls, originally trained as a psychiatric social worker, marriage and family counselor, and psychotherapist. Her personal experiences in childbirth and new motherhood led to her doctoral research, developing self-help programs where experienced mothers helped expectant ones with candid information and emotional support. That work provided the philosophical foundation for this book.

Since completing her doctorate, Dr. Feldman has taught psychology and women's studies at Hofstra and New York universities. She has cohosted television shows offering mental and physical health information to women of all ages. For two years, she hosted her own television program, called "The Art of Mental Health," which focused on the importance of providing emotional support in all the service professions.

Dr. Feldman combines her interest in psychology with writing, particularly about the movies. Her psychological film criticism appears regularly in *Human Behavior* magazine and occasionally in *Psychology Today*. She is planning a collection of these reviews.